STRESS AND THE RISK OF PSYCHOBIOLOGICAL DISORDER IN COLLEGE WOMEN

Alfred B. Heilbrun, Jr.

University Press of Ameica, Inc.
Lanham • New York • Oxford

Copyright © 1998 by
University Press of America,® Inc.
4720 Boston Way
Lanham, Maryland 20706

12 Hid's Copse Rd.
Cummor Hill, Oxford OX2 9JJ

Library of Congress Cataloging-in-Publication Data

Heilbrun, Alfred B.
Stress and the risk of psychobiological disorder in college women /
Alfred B. Heilbrun, Jr.
p. cm.
Includes index.
1. Women college students--Mental health. 2. Stress in youth. 3.
Women college students--Diseases. 4. Anorexia nervosa--Etiology.
5. Cardiovascular system--Diseases--Etiology. 6. Type A behavior.
I. Title.
RC451.4.S7H44   1997 616'.001'9--dc21 97-13317 CIP

ISBN 0-7618-0845-0 (cloth: alk. ppr.)
ISBN 0-7618-0846-9 (pbk: alk. ppr.)

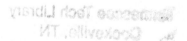

To Marian and our children

who have been responsible

for encouraging my best

efforts as a psychologist

Table of Contents

Preface

Preface

The role of women has undergone considerable revision over the past 20-30 years. This observation is very likely true across all western societies and most certainly true in the United States. Although the revised opportunities and expectations for women have been widely lauded by bookwriters, the media, and social-science researchers, much less attention has been directed at the psychological cost factor if such there is. Although my initial goals were not restricted to the cost issue, I eventually became convinced that the study of stress in college women during the 1980s and 1990s readily attracted that focus. This book on stress and risk of serious psychobiological consequences grew out of a substantial number of studies that were completed within the six-year span I allocated to this line of research.

The stress-research program could not have been completed without the help of students who made their time, effort, talent, and enthusiasm available to me. I would like to extend my special gratitude to Scott Bell, Deborah Bloomfield, Alison Flodin, Michelle Frank, Eric Friedberg, Lisa Friedberg, Ann Harris, Amiee Handfinger, Gwen Hausman, Jordan Karp, Robin Lozman, Kelly Mofield, Constance Mulqueen, Nancy Palchanis, Victoria Pepe, Lauren Putter, Diane Renert, David Salamon, Nancy Witt, Alyson Worobow, and Dawna Wydra. I can only hope that they gained as much from participation as they contributed.

Chapter 1

Stress and Disorder in Competitive Western Societies

Competition in Western Societies

Few would debate the virtues of individual freedom in contemporary America or in other western societies around the world. There is no other form of society that compares with a democracy as far as opportunities for personal attainment and satisfaction are concerned. I am referring here to something more than accommodation to the ordinary expectations imposed by a given society. Rather, the reward of attainment in a free society derives from the pursuit and achievement of individual goals that satisfy personal ambitions and attract the recognition and respect of others. To stand out rather than simply fitting in epitomizes constructive individual striving. The indispensable basis for attainment in a free society is competition which pits individuals against one another for the symbols and substance of success. Important theories of human behavior could be brought to bear in support of this contention, such as Adler's (1929) early emphasis upon superiority striving in explaining psychopathology. However, the role of competitive motivation and behavior in free societies seems self-evident. Only the parameters of competition may be subject to variation from one society to the next.

The rules of competition, as popularly conceived if not practiced, would have boys and girls, men and women, enter into common pursuit of the goals available within a society; achievement of success would be measured by substantive acquisition, assigned status, and personal esteem. However, competitive societies do not guarantee equal success to all who compete or any success at all for that matter, since the essence of competition is the eventual separation of participants into some who win and even more who lose. It makes no difference whether competition is in the interpersonal, educational, work, or play spheres. Some people will do well, more will do less well, and the remainder stand to inherit whatever modest legacies that remain available. It was the uneven rules governing individual competition, especially in the workplace, that fostered much of the ferment provided by the women's movement.

This book is not about the virtues of individual freedom but rather dwells upon the casualties of competition in contemporary American society. Women, now offered a much fairer opportunity to compete with men, must contend with a level of stress equivalent to that long endured by ambitious males, if not greater. The question I will entertain is whether the increments of stress from success-oriented competition increases the risk of psychobiological disorder in the American woman. These are not the casualties of competition that readily come to mind in the American free enterprise system. We hear more about those who are not equipped to compete and fail along the way because they lack talent, motivation, or culturally-bound opportunity. The targets of my concern in this book are young-adult women who have assets that promise some degree of attainment in our culture -- intelligence, the opportunity for higher education, white majority status, and the success orientation that derives from a middle-class background. Despite these seeming advantages, the critical subjects under investigation find themselves contending with severe stress which they are seemingly unable to manage very effectively. Bombarded by stress, these women expose themselves to the risk of serious physical dysfunction as the normal mechanisms for maintaining bodily integrity are compromised. The multifaceted risks facing young-adult college women under stress represent one important reason why females became the focal research interest rather than males.

The reality of heavy stress and the risk of stress-related psychobiological disorder do not exhaust the varied psychological costs of the competitive system by any means, and this book does not pretend to offer a complete picture of the downside of competition once engaged. Furthermore, I shall not address the various pitfalls that disqualify otherwise promising women (and men) who never make it out of the starting gate as far as pursuing success is concerned. Drugs, alcohol, school dropout, social alienation, and crime are readily identifiable as diversions from constructive attainment. Less obvious, perhaps, is the siphoning effect of vicarious achievement upon individual motivation gained through the success of public luminaries. The veneration of highly publicized and grossly overpaid athletes and entertainers by their fans may diminish the importance of their own personal attainment through competition, although which comes first could be debated. Attaining success in the particular ways condoned by the broader society requires talent and sustained effort over long periods of time, and even then individual chances are not that great. Being confronted by intolerable stress or other diversions may make the odds for success even longer and the chances for maladjustment or disorder that much greater.

The point being made here is that individual freedom to compete may involve a serious risk to those who accept the challenge but cannot keep pace in the race for success or who choose not to even try despite apparent assets. This is not the stuff emphasized by high school civics classes, where, understandably, positive encouragement to take on the formidable challenges of successful adulthood is more likely to be encountered. Tokens of success, popularly conceived, are less controversial motivators than the costs of failure.

Social Philosophy and the Scientific Explanation of Disorder

Individual freedom within a society not only provides a context for competitive efforts to achieve but also promotes diverse social/political philosophies regarding the role of that society in determining the outcome of competition. One philosophic distinction that is commonly applied to the role of society in determining individual attainment is "conservative" versus "liberal," although these labels are used to distinguish a far-broader range of social and political alternatives. The conservative view, as applied to success of the individual, would hold that the state should play a minimal role in determining whether someone competes effectively, especially in the career sense. Winning or losing in this competition should be a matter of individual responsibility; success should depend upon who has higher motivation, who has more talent, who is better able to learn. A liberal view would emphasize the role of some collective entity and its responsibility for the betterment of those individuals within its sphere of authority. A larger body, such as the state or nation, insures the fairness of competition for achieving social goals. More than that, it may intervene in an effort to influence the outcome of competition and to improve the fortunes of those whose opportunity to be successful has been obstructed. Conservative-versus-liberal may be an overused contrast in philosophies, but the difference in emphasis upon individual responsibility is relevant to the concern of this book -- examining the risk of stress-related disorders in college women.

There are several approaches to explaining the risk of behavioral disorders scientifically, and these options bear a relationship to social philosophy in my way of thinking. Most of these alternatives share a biological slant. Disorder may follow from contamination by a foreign intruder into the body (e.g., a microorganism or toxic substance). General paresis, for example, involves severe behavioral symptoms such as delusions and results from an inflammation of the brain caused by the invading spirochaete syphilis (Cameron, 1963). Central nervous system anomalies have been linked to forms of schizophrenia as when Crow (1980, 1985) proposed a Type I schizophrenia based upon neurochemical imbalance and a Type II schizophrenia that comes from abnormal brain structure. Faulty genetic endowment has attracted its share of attention as an antecedent to serious psychopathology as well (Gottesman, McGuffin, & Farmer, 1987). For the most part, biological explanations minimize the responsibility of the individual in the development of disorder. Rather, the individual is readily cast as the victim of conditions that are beyond personal control.

An alternative to biological explanation of disorder is found in the belief that maladaptive behaviors are learned. Serious disorder evolves from these acquired maladaptive behaviors compounded by the person's efforts to deal with their effects, efforts that sometimes make matters worse. Explanations in learning terms are more likely to emphasize individual responsibility for symptom development. People may be viewed as their own worst enemies as they become increasingly mired in their conflicts, frustrations, procrastinations, and self-defeating efforts to compensate for the satisfactions that are so obviously missing in their lives. This book will consider the risk factors for three stress-related disorders in women, and they will attract explanation in learning terms. The risk factors will represent a variety of personality traits that at some point have been acquired through experience, either before or after stress became a burden. In other words, these traits may have been instrumental in mobilizing stress to problematic levels or may represent a response to stress. In either case, learned personality factors combine with stress to provide a risk of psychobiological disorder.

It may seem odd to entwine social philosophy and scientific explanation of abnormal behavior, since the former is a matter of belief and the latter is ostensibly a product of scientific evidence. However, it should be kept in mind that there remains a wide gap between the evidence and the explanation of psychopathology, and there is ample opportunity for philosophic bias to intrude into the scientific process. Many choose to believe that individuals are generally not to be held accountable for behavioral disorders, very much in keeping with a liberal philosophy. I start with a different set of assumptions. The origins of the stress-related disorders considered in this book are to be found in the woman's learning experiences. As she grapples with the competitive demands of a culture steeped in the success ethic, conflicts arise and unfortunate choices are made that expose her to chronic stress and, in the long run, to the risk of serious compromise of body integrity. In the final analysis, people are responsible for their individual dilemmas and for the failure to correct them.

To contend that we are responsible for the stress we suffer and for the disordered behavior that may follow in its wake may seem lacking in compassion for those who are psychobiologically troubled. While such an extreme view might be an antidote to the current trend toward assigning responsibility to imperfections in neural tissue or genetic endowment, I feel a learning view of psychopathology is not that unsympathetic. It is not that individuals necessarily learn behaviors at discrete points in time that are obviously going to have devastating effects on their psychological health. The future may hold disorder in store for them, because they have no way of knowing that a behavior will be to their long-term detriment. For example, I will consider the woman's perceptual distortion of her body size as a risk factor in the development of anorexia nervosa. Systematic overstatement of body size is a cognitive trait that can contribute to the choice of serious dieting or can transform dieting to obsessive food restraint and semi-starvation after a choice is made. Body-image distortion is also a learned behavior; women are not neurologically or genetically predisposed to view themselves as fatter than they really are. This distortion may go unrecognized by the woman, but despite lack of conscious intent it can have serious psychological implications. People, like the woman at anorectic risk, are responsible for adopting the behaviors that make them vulnerable to a given disorder. However, they should be held less accountable for their failure to appreciate that these choices place them at-risk.

Massive efforts to educate children and adults regarding the dangers of drugs, alcohol, and tobacco make it difficult to claim that the decision to use them is ever reached without having been made aware of the risk involved. There is nothing comparable designed to educate girls about the dangers of eating restraint or overreacting to menstruation. Few warnings are posted to inform young women of America that unrestrained competitiveness can be hazardous to their health. Even less effort is made to warn the vulnerable among them that they should be especially cautious about specific behavioral choices. Nothing malicious about this; there just has not been a coherent and compelling message available regarding the psychological risk factors in stress-related disorder to pass along to females who might be at-risk.

The Meaning of Stress and Its Relationship to Disorder

Stress refers to a response or state of an individual. It is aroused from stimulation in the environment that generally signals danger or from the person's own mental representations of threat. Provocative stimulation is itself sometimes called stress, so to avoid confusion the term "stressors" will be used to refer to cues, extrinsic or intrinsic, that elicit stress responses. The stress state is comprised of two components. One is a mental component that involves awareness at some level that something (the stressor) threatens the person's wellbeing. The other is a biological component involving the autonomic nervous system that is activated when threat is experienced. The effects of autonomic arousal are largely responsible for the symptoms of a stress state. These indicators of stress are readily recognized -- nervousness, pounding heart, excessive sweating, etc. Stress is usually experienced as unpleasant by most people, and they will be motivated to alleviate the unpleasantness whenever possible. There are varying degrees of stress tolerance shown by individuals, however, and even a few people who seem to thrive on stress and a "stirred-up" state. There are no universal truths regarding human behavior, but that people seek to escape from the unpleasantness of a stress state comes close.

Given this brief exposition of stress as a response, several further points require elaboration before moving on. We might first examine the nature of threat that instigates the stress response and the myriad ways in which people try to alleviate stress (see Lazarus and Folkman, 1984, for a more extended discussion). Threat should be considered a matter of interpretation; whether something menaces personal wellbeing depends upon how the person perceives that stimulus and what

represents wellbeing. This introduces considerable room for subjectivity into who experiences stress and how much. The personal
stamp placed upon threat is especially obvious in social relationships,
because they can be remarkably complicated and open to variable interpretation. There would be clearcut consensus regarding the danger of a
large bear encountered in the wild; far more variation in perceived
threat would be expected given a first-date social encounter.

Relief from stress based upon actions taken by the stressed individual is separated into two types (Lazarus & Folkman, 1984). Direct
actions are addressed to whatever is perceived as the actual source of
stress. Coping with stress in this way is generally deemed to be the
most effective, since successful coping can permanently remove the
source of stress or at least reduce stressor impact to a tolerable level.
However, the pitfalls of direct coping are not difficult to identify. The
person may misrepresent the source of stress, may select an
inappropriate action that fails to change the stressor for the better, or
may have no direct recourse available.

If direct coping proves to be a problem, indirect actions are available. These do not influence the source of stress but, instead,
temporarily relieve the unpleasant emotions of the stress state. Sometimes the stressor is a temporary phenomenon and disappears on its
own; in the meantime, indirect coping makes life more comfortable.
Paramount among the indirect coping strategies are the ever-available
psychological defenses. These allow the person to evade the threatening qualities of the stressor, if only for awhile, by putting the stressor
out of mind or revising what it means and thereby reducing its threatening qualities. The bad news about the defenses is that they never
change the objective reality of a stressor. In fact, they may prove harmful in some cases by delaying or even preventing direct actions that
otherwise might be taken to remove a source of stress. The good news
is that defensiveness and other indirect means of coping with the emotions of stress are readily available and can make difficult situations
more bearable. Direct and indirect action are not mutually exclusive
tactics for stress reduction. Indirect means of coping with the emotions
of stress may accompany efforts to deal directly with a stressor.

Stress, Cognition, and Disorder

The cognitive processes will be at the heart of my discussion of
stress and the risk of disorder found later in this book. Some acknowledgement regarding how cognition is to be treated seems imperative,

since so much has been written on the subject that is extraneous to my concern. First, I shall deal with the cognitive processes from a personality perspective as a researcher interested in individual cognitive traits. This interest in how people vary in psychological structure will depart from the mainstream concern of the cognitive scientist committed to understanding how psychological systems work across people (the nature of memory, attention, perception, etc.). The specific implications of this choice shall be discussed in the next chapter.

Secondly, I shall consider cognition in as simple a manner as its complex nature allows. My goal is to describe cognition and the various processes subsumed under this category of behavior in ways that are meaningful to the intended readership of this book and (hopefully) not objectionable to the scientific purist. To begin with, cognition for me refers to the mental phenomena that play such a critical role in human behavior, directing activities from the most trivial to the most complex, the most deplorable to the most praiseworthy. The mind allows us to produce art, create national policy, or make scientific discoveries; mental processes are equally responsible for brutal street crimes, acts of terrorism, and psychological disorders.

Cognition includes mental activities that make it possible to utilize information available to us from the outside environment or from within ourselves. These activities are generally well known, since they represent obvious ways that information must be treated before it can serve as the basis for action. Attention refers to the process that controls sampling of stimulation from our surroundings or from within; awareness of stimulation makes it available for subsequent action. Some stimulation has immediate meaning to us, whereas other stimulation that registers requires interpretation before it becomes meaningful. The process by which the person assigns meaning to stimulation is called perception. Information, as meaningful stimulation, is processed in any number of ways. We make judgments based upon information; we withdraw information from memory store; we catalogue evaluative statements and make reference to them as values; we reason by drawing associations between pieces of information; we plan by projecting future action contingent upon current information; we defend ourselves by distorting information so that it is less distressing, at least for awhile. There are innumerable other mental processes that make use of information gained through attention and perception. Cognition from a personality standpoint directs our interest to how an individual systematically attends to her environment, assigns meaning to stimulation that registers, and processes this information as a prelude to action, all relative to others.

The risk of progression from stress to disorder, emphasizing the role of cognitive personality traits, shall involve certain assumptions. In most general terms, it will be assumed that women come to experience excessive stress, allow it to continue, and succumb to psychobiological disorder if they display certain personality characteristics. These risk-conferring traits may be instrumental in provoking and maintaining stress in the first place or may be part of an ineffective coping process that adds to the chances of a disordered outcome. Moreover, the personality traits may be quite innocuous in themselves so that someone with these characteristics but without elevated stress would not be penalized by their presence. By the same token, if a woman were under stress but did not share these particular characteristics, her risk of disorder would be diminished.

Women College Students as Objects of Study

My initial interest in stress and the risk of disorder in college students was not restricted to women. Thirty years of experience with college mental health agencies had led me to assume that stress was not only a common commodity on campuses but one that was shared by male and female students alike. These assumptions have not changed, but experience with mounting a program of research into stress and the risk of disorder encouraged me to slant investigation toward the college woman. One reason had to do with the practical logistics of research. My early formulations and the method chosen to investigate stress and its health risks required that I find dependable measures capable of disclosing early symptoms of serious psychobiological disorder. The options were more numerous for women than men and offered greater latitude for investigation. Why standardized inquiries into body-related health problems for women were more available is difficult to say. It could result from something as important as a greater female somatic vulnerability to disorder, particularly in response to stress, or something as unremarkable as the personal interests of test developers.

The choice of women as the primary object of study was predicated upon interest as well as practical convenience, however. It became increasingly evident that the relationships between ambition and stress for the young-adult women I studied were more complicated than was true for her male counterpart. The added complications made the research more intriguing. They also made it likely that any effort to extrapolate the cost of ambition from the male experience would provide an imperfect fit for the woman as she confronted alternatives in her selection of long-range goals involving career and family. Men, because of gender-role prescriptions that have remained intact despite the social ferment of the past 2-3 decades, are expected to work and maintain a family. There is stress associated with fulfilling these expectations, more for some men than others depending upon self-confidence, level of aspiration, and competition associated with chosen goals. With women, as I shall elaborate later, stress evolves not only from uncertainties and competition in achieving goals but conflict between goals.

Why were college students chosen as the object of research? After years of enlisting these students in my investigations as a matter of practical research necessity, the time finally arrived when such subjects were in principle the subject of choice. For one thing, I needed a population of subjects who would, without much exception, entertain lofty ambitions and for whom the satisfaction of these goals still lay ahead. For another, they should be no stranger to competition as the basis for pursuing their ambitions. High levels of stress had to be represented in the subject population, and, as I have said, this commodity is not in short supply among college students. Finally, research involving risk of disorder from current stress requires subjects who are old enough to be realistically considered as candidates for future disorder but young enough to be still functioning within normal psychobiological limits. The research program was concerned with future risk and not with current clinical conditions. Although we did not screen the thousands of subjects in the program by a rigorous diagnostic procedure, I am convinced that only a small percentage presented the full-blown psychobiological disorder that was being investigated.

A Proposed Paradigm for Stress and the Risk of Stress-related Disorder

The general explanatory framework for the risk of stress-related disorder grew out of three distinct programs of research. Each line of research considered the combined presence of stress, various personality factors, and early symptoms of potentially serious psychobiological disorder. It was not assumed at the outset that all programs of investigation would be embraced within a single broad proposal regarding the risk of psychobiological dysfunction posed by stress. In fact, the chances of a common explanation seemed dim. The symptom pictures for each disorder varied widely, the timetables for stress effects upon the body were not synchronous, and gender-relevance varied widely across disorders.

Premenstrual syndrome (PMS)/dysmenorrhea, disorders of menstruation, are restricted to women and anorexia nervosa nearly so. Disordered menstruation and obsessive restraint of eating represent clinical conditions in which the body comes to be compromised in very different ways with symptom patterns that show little commonality. In addition, the period of transition from predisposing heavy stress to dysfunctional body condition is likely to be short-term (anorexia) or intermediate-term (PMS) in duration as gauged by the ages at which the disorder commonly appears. There seems to be little common-ground between these disorders save their special relevance to women.

Exploring the risk of cardiovascular problems as a stress-related phenomenon had even less in common with the parallel inquiries into menstrual problems and anorexia nervosa than they had with each other. Investigation had to be based upon a different strategy, since cardiovascular problems are not likely to be manifest for several years from the time peak stress is recorded in our research. In this program of research, long-term risk was inferred in part from the presence of a personality style that has received considerable attention as a stress-related antecedent to coronary heart disease. The Type A personality, hard-driven and ambitious to the point of obsession, is believed to be a dangerous prelude to future cardiovascular problems as unremitting stress is maintained at high levels. For us, Type A status substituted as a mediating stage with cardiovascular dysfunction being the long-range risk. In a sense, Type A behaviors represented an early symptom picture just as menstrual discomfort and budding anorectic characteristics served as early warning signs of disorder. Since Type A status and cardiovascular problems are common to both women and men, this line of research was appropriate for both sexes. College men were included as controls along with the usual women subjects in order to answer questions about the comparability of stress, personality, and risk factors across gender lines.

The explanatory paradigm of stress-related disorder for women in a competitive society, evolving from the three disparate programs of research, begins with the assumption that individual attainment as an adult female can fall within either or both of two general domains. The woman may achieve in a career sense or she may achieve in an interpersonal sense. Career achievement is based upon competition in a more obvious way. Success here is defined by popularly-recognized symbols such as grades in school and wages and job status in the workplace. Career success is also confirmed by the deference and respect of other people or by positive self-evaluation.

Interpersonal achievement elicits its own brand of competition in which women vie for acquaintances, friends, sexual liaisons, and marital relationships that provide opportunity for children. Here the competition may be less obvious, but striving for popularity, intimacy, and successful social bonds goes well beyond a passive sense of destiny. Women compare themselves and are compared with others concerning their popularity, sexual attractiveness, social competence, and quality of friendships and marriage. Achieving these interpersonal goals not only helps to establish social status in the eyes of others but assumes critical importance in defining personal identity. These observations apply to men as well, but a legacy from the traditional role accorded to women would stamp interpersonal accomplishment as a more paramount concern for them. In my view, these interpersonal goals can be pursued by the woman in the same competitive way as is true for career accomplishment; popularity, good friendships and successful marriage are available to only some and are open to contest.

Considering two types of attainment, career and interpersonal, extends the opportunity for success. This qualifies as true for women as long as they can achieve in both the career and interpersonal domains. However, what if career-oriented women, as we would expect to find in the college ranks, cannot succeed in one way without being penalized in achieving their goals in the other? Even worse, the college woman may believe that success in one realm actually precludes success in the other. Either way, the woman could be faced with a sense of lost opportunity and failed obligation. If the person is a young-adult woman about 18 years old, like most of those studied in our programs of research, this sense of conflict could translate into a dismaying view of the future and compound the stress normally attending competition for difficult goals.

Given a burden of stress that becomes intolerable, those women who project themselves as in danger of losing the competition for career and/or interpersonal success may try to compensate by selecting some substitute goal that seems more attainable or by elevating their efforts toward the standard goals of society. Compensation by substituting a new goal for those in seeming conflict or by increasing competitive fervor may succeed up to a point. Dieting may provide a slimmer body to the pre-anorectic or the obsessive competitiveness and striving of the

Type A may accrue the tokens of academic success. Eventually, body thinness, given an anorectic solution to conflict, will become a source of stress in itself as dieting assumes a compulsive quality and ingestion of food becomes aversive. Thus, the stress level of the female may not be reduced even though she makes progress toward the substitute goal of body thinness. The hypercompetitive solution to achievement concerns of the Type A woman also fails to curtail stress because of the distressing nature of competition itself. In either case, the risk of eventual harm to the body resides in the attempt to resolve discomforting dilemmas of achievement by the choice of behaviors that do not resolve stress and actually may add to the burden.

The risk involved in the case of menstrual impairment is to some extent contingent upon biological predisposition, and this sets it apart from the vulnerability picture that will be developed for anorexia nervosa and cardiovascular disease. Although I will draw upon the dynamics of achievement in the college woman as a way of explaining one set of risk factors that were discovered, menstrual dysfunction will depend less upon this source of explanation than will be true for the other stress-related disorders.

Compensation by anorectic goal substitution or escalated Type A competitiveness, as well as increasing dysfunction of a vulnerable menstrual system, will more likely appear as a response to stress if the woman demonstrates certain types of cognitive or social traits. The personality characteristics prove detrimental and pose a special risk, because they facilitate the progression toward serious psychobiological disorder. These traits can be maladaptive to the extent that they foster the behavioral excesses that constitute these disorders.

Given a continuation of heavy stress and its maladaptive effects, body integrity may eventually be compromised. This could result from the ill-effects of semi-starvation following all-too-successful dieting that merges into phobic disengagement from eating (anorexia nervosa). Strain on the cardiovascular system given chronic stress from unrelenting competition and unrequited ambition (Type A pattern) could have an eroding effect. Problems within the menstrual cycle could deteriorate into disabling symptoms of disorder as stress and personality combine to promote distress.

This proposed paradigm elaborating the risk of psychologically-mediated somatic disorders remains to be confirmed by forthcoming evidence in the chapters to follow. Perhaps "confirmed" is too strong a term to use in this instance, since the research was geared to isolate hypothetical vulnerability factors for each disorder and not to provide critical tests of the underlying theory of ambition-driven stress. You will be provided a large number of empirically-documented risk factors associated with the three stress-related disorders under consideration. It is possible that a different explanation for why these factors emerged may be more compelling, or you may prefer to adopt a more empirical view and consider risk markers without concerning yourself with understanding why these particular psychological variables were found. I have introduced my own stress-and-personality paradigm based upon ambition and competition for goals on the assumption that this explanation might lend further authenticity to the evidence disclosed by our research.   It is one thing to report risk factors confirmed by statistics but something more to show that they can be integrated.

Chapter 2

Methodology Issues in Studying Stress and the Risk of Disordered Behavior

This chapter will be concerned with the methodology used in our programs of research. Stark description of these procedures without elaboration would not be satisfactory, since the manner in which psychopathology research is conducted varies widely and is replete with controversy. Choices I have made regarding how to investigate risk of disorder are best understood within the context of the issues that divide investigators. There is something to be gained from considering scientific method even if the emphasis in this book will be on the professional and practical implications of the evidence. At a time when understanding of dysfunctional development still remains rudimentary, the methodology by which evidence is generated may have much to say about what represents important increments to our knowledge. Readers, whether they are mental health professionals, scientists, or the lay public, should take the time to consider these research issues.

Inquiry into the Development of Disorder: The Search for Risk Factors Rather than Causal Antecedents

One of the common bonds among researchers into psychopathology is the belief that someday our efforts will pay off in the discovery of what causes human psychological or psychobiological disorders. As the causes of disorder are isolated, the possibilities for prevention are greatly enhanced. Rather than taking belated action in which we attempt to ameliorate the symptoms of disorder after they appear, recognition of causes makes it more possible to circumvent problems before they start by directing attention to their sources. Progress into discovering causal antecedents is impeded by the serious difficulties facing this kind of developmental research, however. Some of these difficulties are technical, having to do with the logistical dilemma brought about by the attempt to study conditions prevailing before the fact of disorder has been established. The dilemma is two-fold. How do you go back into peoples' lives after they have come to suffer from a particular disorder in order to discover what conditions prevailed at some critical earlier period? If this challenge were not enough, how is it possible to prove beyond reasonable doubt that a given prevailing condition contributed in a cause-and-effect manner to developing the disorder?

The technical challenges to causal research are accompanied by another problem that slows our progress. The vague uncertainties of our state of knowledge regarding why some people succumb to psychological disorder provide a breeding ground for speculation. Advocates from various theoretical camps, whether they emphasize learned behavior, genetics, neurological impairment, or social-cultural impact, may prove unreceptive to disclosures relating to cause that favor approaches other than their own. Since the nature of evidence bearing upon psychopathogenesis inevitably falls short of being compelling, there is little to dislodge the scientists from their particular theoretical positions. That is one reason why I am addressing this book to the professional or the informed public. Their concerns and responsibilities have much more to do with the unfortunate results of stress and how to detect the danger of serious psychobiological disorder than with allegiance to particular explanatory viewpoints.

If I was not always wise enough to avoid the pitfalls of assuming I was engaged in causal research into stress and disorder, I am now. The term "cause" is one I will avoid as our research is discussed. Rather, I will talk about "risk factors," behaviors that signal the danger ahead of a particular disorder. Risk will be assumed when an association is demonstrated between a psychological factor and the early warning signs of any given stress-related disorder -- high stress and the beginning symptoms defining that disorder.

These risk factors, taken individually or in combination, are geared to anticipate a particular stress-driven disorder that may loom ahead. Some of these risk factors might be considered part of the causal dynamics of disorder. However, it will not be my mission to argue for that conclusion no matter what my personal convictions might be. The research programs were never geared to proving that one thing leads to another; correlational research never does.

As I shall discuss at greater length and with examples a few pages ahead, risk factors are considered to be signposts that point toward a given disordered psychobiological outcome. They do not imply inevitability nor necessarily a cause-and-effect relation with disorder. The stronger the signs and the more signs that are in evidence, the higher the risk of a particular disordered outcome is presumed to be. Less intense markers of risk or their diminished number offer the opposite expectation.

Having spent this much time in relinquishing claim to causal explanation by the research evidence ahead, I must acknowledge that this more conservative position bears only upon assumption of proof. I found it impossible to write about the risk of psychobiological stress disorder without attempting to put the empirical findings in some sort of understandable context. In fact, I have already begun this process in the first chapter when the assumptions regarding competition and achievement were presented. These assumptions play a prominent role in understanding why the risk factors contribute to pathogenesis. This sounds like causal attribution, and perhaps it is. The difference for me is that I do not consider the evidence at hand as proof of these dynamic explanations; logic and common sense are called for in weighing their worth. As I have said before, readers are free to invoke their own interpretations or to simply use the risk factors as empirically-verified signposts that warn of impending disorder in women.

<u>Advantages and limitations of current research practices in</u> <u>studying the origins of disorder</u>. Reference has been made to the availability of several scientific procedures that have been used in the effort to understand why human behavior becomes disordered. I shall describe these as succinctly as possible and comment upon the more obvious advantages and liabilities intrinsic to each. This review will hopefully make clear why a new at-risk methodology for studying psychobiological dysfunction was devised rather than depending upon existing procedures.

One major obstacle complicating causal research into the origins of psychopathology has to do with the substantial time lapse between the clearcut emergence of a disorder and the earlier conditions that might be critical to its development. Added to this problem is the low base rate for any given disorder (e.g., 1 in 100 people in the general population will be diagnosed as schizophrenic) that may complicate sampling procedures. The complexity of causal antecedents, including their interactive qualities, may or may not present a problem depending upon the premise of investigation. If a faulty genetic structure is assumed to be responsible for a given disorder, the issue of complexity may not loom large. If antecedent interest is focused on some disorder in which learning plays a major role, the complications of interdependent behaviors introduce a special challenge. Research procedures in causal research differ in large measure because they try to circumvent these obstacles in different ways, doing so with more or less success. What is available in way of resources account for the remaining differences.

We can start with the research approach that is generally acknowledged to be the best basis for discovering the roots of psychopathology. Longitudinal investigation seeks the origins of disorder by following the same people over a substantial period of time. The results of observation and measurement at the beginning of the period of study will eventually be compared to data collected later, and formulations regarding preclinical status, change, and outcome can be derived. Ideally, the tracking period for longitudinal research bearing upon causation not only should begin prior to the appearance of clinical disorder but before critical developmental events may be in evidence. Tracking should continue until disorder is confirmed for those who prove to be vulnerable.

The potential advantage of longitudinal study is clear and compelling. The scientist can derive a more definitive picture of how a disorder develops if the same people are studied from premorbidity to morbidity. To the extent that information relevant to causation is recorded from the outset, following the same people over time should provide clues to the origins of disorder. I have considered the drawbacks to the longitudinal method in studying the causes of disorder before (Heilbrun, 1973). The logistics of longitudinal study are very costly, well beyond the resources of the ordinary researcher. Investigation that requires tracking the same individuals over time must contend with the attrition of subjects. Are the subjects who remain comparable to those who drop from the study? Longitudinal investigation of the same individuals often involves repeated contact with subjects; effects generated by repeated observation can be difficult to disentangle from the ordinary life experiences being studied.

The value of longitudinal study, no matter how well orchestrated from a logistical perspective, depends upon the quality of conception and the measurement technology that mark its beginning. If a researcher overlooks the importance of a particular variable at the outset and does not collect relevant data, it may not be possible to correct this oversight later. Even the initial inclusion of a critical variable goes for naught if the original measure proves to be flawed. A second chance with improved measurement procedures may not be feasible. Thus, undeniable advantage of following the same person over time is lost if the wrong questions are posed at the outset or if poor measures are used to generate information.

The longitudinal method, taken alone, is not a responsive technique for answering questions about the origins of disorder. The researcher launching a longitudinal investigation cannot be expected to raise important questions at the outset to the extent that they depend upon yet undiscovered evidence. When the problem of why a given disorder develops is complex, a premium is placed upon discovery as a prelude to further investigation and programmatic research is called for. Longitudinal study does not lend itself to programmed research, since the time consumed is prohibitive. In my opinion, longitudinal research into antecedents of disorder is most valuable toward the end of the discovery process when definitive confirmation of a well-articulated theory is required.

Finally, longitudinal research into the development of disorder is rendered impractical when the target is a low base rate disorder. This problem received special attention in the 1970s and 1980s when "high-risk" longitudinal study of antecedents to schizophrenia was proposed using the children of a diagnosed schizophrenic parent as subjects (e.g., Mednick & Schulsinger, 1970). The base rate of schizophrenia, often cited as 1 in 100 within the general population, made random sampling from that population unfeasible as a source of premorbid subjects for longitudinal study. In principle, 100 subjects would have to be tracked in order to establish the antecedents of 1 followed through to eventual schizophrenia. Genetic family-history research indicated that by selecting the children of a schizophrenic parent for longitudinal study, the base rate for schizophrenia would be raised to 10-15 for 100 subjects sampled. Thus, "high-risk" investigation was supposed to provide the advantage of the longitudinal method but keep subject numbers within reason.

Unfortunately, the "high-risk" procedure may have confounded methodology with results. If, as many would argue, there are multiple contributions to schizophrenia, including genetic, this methodological approach would certainly emphasize the importance of heredity out of proportion to its merit. What explanation for the disorder other than heredity could be expected to receive support if the basis for subject selection is genetic predisposition to schizophrenia as defined by a parental history of that disorder?

Laboratory study of disordered development should guarantee better control of the conditions under which data are collected from subjects. Better control, in turn, may allow the scientist to detect relationships that would be elusive given a less precise method of gathering evidence. The laboratory method, while useful for some types of psychological research, has not been of great value in studying antecedents of psychopathology. Laboratory experimentation is ideally suited for revealing cause-and-effect relationships, but the advantage of added precision is compromised by the complicated dynamics of clinical disorders. The problem, of course, is that it is nearly impossible to devise experimental models to be tested in the laboratory that can meet both the requirements of rigorous scientific control, on the one hand, and simulate the involved dynamics of incipient disorder on the other. Laboratory study of questions relating to developmental psychopathology does have value. However, it lies in the controlled analysis of specific elements within a broader explanatory model.

Cross-sectional investigation represents a less demanding alternative to the longitudinal method from a logistical perspective. Rather than following the same individuals over long time periods, cross-sectional investigation involves collecting independent samples of subjects from some larger population to test different hypotheses concerning faulty development. The major advantage of the cross-sectional method is the flexibility accorded to the researcher in considering new questions that evolve from completed studies. This represents a priority requirement when complicated behavioral issues are at stake. Programmatic research makes it possible to devise new studies in which you build upon the revelations of earlier ones in the program. A cross-sectional methodology allows you to generate the new samples that can be used for these unanticipated studies using subjects comparable to those included in earlier investigations. This partnership between programmed research and a cross-sectional methodology was exploited to gather the evidence described in subsequent chapters.

The problems of cross-sectional research in studying the developmental origins of psychopathology have much to do with the appropriateness of the subjects that are sampled. If subjects are to be relevant targets of investigation who can provide evidence regarding the origins of a particular disorder, they must share characteristics that would make them vulnerable to that disorder -- gender, age, social demographics, etc. The cross-sectional approach to data collection obviously lacks the advantage of extended observation over time. This will mean that a final verdict regarding disorder will not be available to cross-sectional researchers whether they are pursuing causation or isolating risk factors.

The retrospective method for studying developmental disorder depends upon the reconstruction of earlier development through memory. Often it is the disordered person recalling his or her own past that represents the source of data, but family, friends, or anyone else knowing something about the person or the conditions of development also can serve as informants. Just as the longitudinal method is the most revered research strategy among developmental scientists, even though it is infrequently used, the retrospective method is most often the object of ridicule. The major reason that retrospection is disavowed for establishing past events is simple enough; the information is believed to lack authenticity. Either people's memories are not sufficiently reliable to trust what is remembered, or, if memory is not a problem, the person's rendition of the past may be biased.

The basic value of retrospection, paradoxically, is related to a criticism of the method as vulnerable to subjective revision of memories. Even if the limitations of memory do not preclude accurate retrospection, cognitive distortions may detract from the realistic quality of long-term memories, as I have said. Perhaps you will remember only positive things about yourself or others, for example, or just the opposite tendency may prevail. This type of pervasive influence upon memory will no doubt compromise the accuracy of information that is reinstated. However, a second possibility comes to mind that promotes subjectivity of memory to a more valued position. Retrospection may offer the subject an opportunity to accurately report prior events as they were experienced without concern about what actually happened. Unless memory departs radically from the original subjective experience, there is much to be learned from the subjective impressions of the person. Human behavior is contingent largely upon our own interpretation of reality (perception). A retrospective approach to earlier experience may allow the researcher to gain access to important versions of reality that have been instrumental in shaping disordered behavior (Heilbrun, 1971).

Sometimes a researcher may gain access to stored information in clinic files, school records, or in other sources of archival data that seem relevant to eventual disorder. Such file research can offer valuable insight into why some people came to suffer from disorder and others enjoy healthy development. Robins' (1966) investigation into the origins of sociopathic personality is an example of how information in clinic files may prove to be revealing many years later.

It seems fair to say that an important developmental discovery by means of a stored-information strategy of research would have to be somewhat fortuitous. Stored information is static, by definition; what you find is what you get. If the scientist happens to be interested in questions that can be answered by stored information, all well and good. If not or if new questions arise, the limitations of static data soon will be apparent.

Obviously, the source of stored information and the complete-ness of the file will make a great differences in developmental studies of disorder. Complete files maintained in a mental health center offer greater promise of identifying precursors of psychological disorder than school records that emphasize educational factors.

Constituting at-risk groups from a normal population in the study of disordered development. My own efforts to cast light upon the risk of serious psychobiological disorder in college women under heavy stress have depended upon a strategy of research that was devised espe-cially for this program of investigation. This strategy departs from the procedures described over the previous several pages in some ways but shares common features as well. Since the credibility of my findings will depend in part upon the legitimacy of the research procedures gen-erating the evidence, I shall offer a detailed account of the at-risk method.

All developmental psychopathologists are faced with a simple truth; within a normal population there are some who one day will show a particular disorder. If only it were possible to look into the future so that those who are destined to suffer from a particular disorder could be identified at an earlier period when they were functioning within normal limits. Given such an option, the researcher would have an invaluable opportunity to study the factors associated with the onset of that disorder at a time when pathogenesis is in its beginning stages. In its own way, the at-risk research methodology represents an effort to create just such an opportunity. Seemingly normal subjects are identified who at least stand a chance of demonstrating a particular disorder. Comparison of these at-risk individuals with their peers allows for the discovery of additional risk factors that may be operative in the vulnerable group.

The at-risk method for investigating the antecedents of disorder within a normal population, in our case college females, can be applied with a more immediate and readily satisfied purpose in mind or with a more long-term and demanding goal ahead. By beginning with the basic components of incipient disorder, associated factors can be discovered that would allow you to narrow down which subjects stand a greater chance of eventually demonstrating the symptomatology of a given disorder at a clinical level. In our research programs the "basic components" included a high degree of stress and the presence of subclinical symptoms of a disorder. The identification of associated personality factors that followed should have immediate practical importance, since it provides an early-warning system for trouble to come and allows opportunity for preventive behavioral change.

A more ambitious long-range goal for the at-risk method would involve the use of associated factors to identify subjects at high and low risk for more intense investigation. Research into the early development of a disorder should then be possible as risk factors are considered in terms of causal dynamics and new factors are sought. Our research was geared to reach the more attainable goal -- to confirm the presence of risk factors among college women that warn of disorder ahead.

The selection of risk factors for investigation bears obvious importance, since the wrong choice guarantees wasted research effort. The strategy of choice in our at-risk programs was to seek variables that seemed related to the stress-related disorder in question or to the explanatory context of competition and achievement within which the findings were to be embedded. Some examples might be useful. A major behavioral symptom of the clinical disorder in question attracted research attention if it were amenable to measurement at a subclinical level. The distorted body-imaging found in women suffering from anorexia nervosa is a case in point; varying levels of distortion can be readily identified in a normal population of women. In addition, any behavior that seemed to have some causal significance (in my mind) for a given disorder attracted attention such as self-preoccupation in the investigation of menstrual dysfunctions. Sex-role variables assumed a prominent position as risk factors in all these at-risk programs, since they qualify as important to the achievement goals of the college woman, her ability to engage in competition, and the stress of uncertain accomplishment.

The power of the at-risk methodology depends in an important way upon the characteristics of the population of normal subjects from which the samples are drawn. I already have addressed this methodological consideration, but further comment is called for as the at-risk method is introduced. Since our research goal was to discover factors that were associated with vulnerability to stress-related disorders, it followed that the population of subjects must have the potential for exhibiting these disorders. The greater the potential, the more suitable the population of subjects for at-risk investigation. The 18-year-old college women we sampled were obtained from a population that was close to ideal as far as appropriate gender, age, college attendance, and social-economic class were concerned. These characteristics satisfied the requirements of subject relevance; a recruitment system on campus made it possible to attract the number of subjects required for the numerous studies that were necessary; and the number of college women under serious stress was evident.

Programmatic Research Versus Single-study Investigation

I may be testing the limits of patience in discussing research methodology for those who have a more vested interest in the evidence ahead and its implications. Despite this, I find that there are two more aspects of our investigative procedures that merit at least brief comment, since both have a bearing upon the credibility of the findings. One of these is the programmatic nature of our research. A program of research is distinguished in the most obvious way by the number of studies that are conducted within a more-or-less specific area of scientific concern by a researcher or a team of researchers. The value of programmatic investigation goes beyond the obvious ethic that more evidence is better than less evidence, however.

For one thing, the fact that one study can serve as a prelude to another almost guarantees that new and important questions will be encountered that might not otherwise surface. Not only will questions arise from preceding research, but commitment to a program makes it more likely that answers will be sought. Programmatic research, then, takes cognizance of the fact that scientific efforts in the social sciences are often more important because of the questions they raise than the answers they provide.

Replication of results is often extolled in social science but rarely practiced. Whether the same results can be obtained if a study is repeated speaks to the reliability of the information provided by research. Reliability becomes a critical concern when the tools of investigation are imprecise or the methodology otherwise allows for the influence of uncontrolled or even unrecognized influences upon results. If the same result can be obtained on a new sample of subjects when the same conditions are introduced, more confidence in the evidence is warranted. That replication is rarely practiced (at least rarely reported) can be explained by the disinterest of psychology journals in publishing research devoted exclusively to that issue. Scientists who depend upon their own research to guide subsequent inquiry may be more inclined to verify prior effects, or in the course of conducting an interlocking series of studies, replication may be a natural consequence of building onto prior results.

Replication of previous findings by repeating the same conditions and obtaining the same results is not the only way in which programmatic research can authenticate evidence. It was not even the most likely source of confidence in the credibility of findings. A program of research should eventually establish a network of evidence within which the meaning of new results will either provide a compelling fit or appear out-of-step and pose a problem for interpretation. Information that dovetails harmoniously with other programmatic scientific evidence should command greater confidence. However, a network of established evidence must exist before this stamp of consistency becomes available.

Questionnaire Data as a Scientific Tool

The at-risk procedure for studying the early-warning signs of disorder in a normal population of college females relied considerably upon standardized questionnaires that inquired into the personal, often private, experience of the subject. Use of self-report test information as a means of understanding people has had a checkered history over the past 50 years, especially as a research option.

Concern regarding the use of questionnaire inquiry is likely to take one of two forms when introduced into the methodology of research. Limits on the availability of information requested by questionnaire items or on the accuracy of information obtained from the subject have been used to challenge the usefulness of test scores. An even more popular critical theme has emphasized the role of test-taking styles as a source of diminished response accuracy and invalid measurement. So-called "response sets" have been proposed in which subjects are pictured as selecting more socially-desirable options, acquiescing to item content unduly or engaging in extravagant denial, selecting the first option among many, etc. -- anything but respond in an honest and straightforward way to item content. For many years the use of self-report questionnaires in research had to be routinely accompanied by reassurance that response styles played no important part in determining test scores. The irony of this seems to have escaped the historians of personality and psychopathology research; the routine denial of response-set effects in published research favors the conclusion that this source of concern was of no great importance to begin with.

The questionnaires that you will encounter in the chapters ahead are primarily behavior rating scales that inquire into the basic elements of at-risk status. One set of rating scales considers various symptoms of stress; three other questionnaires look into the behaviors encountered in the anorectic eating disorder, the symptoms of menstrual dysfunction, or the stress-provoking elements of a Type A personality pattern; further ratings will inquire into biological experiences and cognitive representation of relevant events. Some of these tests have enjoyed wide research usage, whereas others were devised specifically for our programs of study. All approach measurement by presenting item content in a straightforward manner and requiring simple ratings in response. The content always bears upon recent internal happenings or recurrent patterns of behavior about which the subject should be aware and capable of reporting accurately. This information was gained anonymously. The simple truth is that the woman herself is the only one who could offer us insight into matters this personal and private, and there is no reason known to me why her revelations should not be considered valid enough for scientific inquiry at the level of group comparisons.

There is another way of confirming my personal impression that questionnaires, when they were used, provided valid accounts of subject behavior. If the women serving as subjects had no real grasp of their inner happenings or preclinical behaviors or chose not to reveal this knowledge, the chances of discovering anything meaningful from programmatic study would be nil. Investigative probes that come up with nonsensical or irrelevant information cannot provide comprehensive meaning, at least over a substantial number of independent studies. In a real sense, the whole body of evidence within each program of research provides validation for the procedures of its component studies to the extent overall integrity of meaning is achieved.

Readers, then, represent a critical arbiter of quality for our methodology. If the conclusions reached across several studies make collective sense relative to each other, in keeping with logic and clinical sophistication, what are the chances that these conclusions were based upon spurious data?

Chapter 3

The Anorectic Eating Disorder and Background Factors Governing Risk

The research evidence that we have collected bearing upon the risk of anorexia nervosa in college women subject to major stress will be presented in three chapters. This chapter will consider the factors that may predispose some women to abnormal patterns of eating associated with excessive concerns about weight and body size. These background factors are considered first, because they are concerned with preliminary issues that set them apart from our mainstream inquiry into anorectic risk. Their preliminary nature led us to focus less on the role of stress in marking vulnerability to disorder and more on broader questions relating to the parameters of our search. The studies covered will be important in setting the stage for the discovery of stress-related risk factors. The questions to be addressed include why some young-adult women fall back on body concerns and peculiarities of eating when they encounter difficulties? More specifically, why did the risk of one type of eating problem (anorexia nervosa) predominate rather than another (bulimia)? The broader social framework of ambition and competition which guided my search for risk factors also will receive attention.

The critical role of stress as a source of risk in anorexia nervosa will receive attention in chapters 4 and 5. These chapters will concentrate upon specific risk factors which, when combined with high stress and muted symptoms, signal a vulnerability to anorectic development. Risk studies will emphasize the cognitive distortions that are associated with the development of anorexia nervosa along with critical social behaviors that serve as vulnerability indicators. Chapters 4 and 5 will differ from each other by emphasizing new risk factors considered individually in chapter 4 and more complex patterns in chapter 5 that involve new risk variables analyzed in combination.

A reasonable beginning for this section of the book on the risk of anorectic disorder in high-stress college women is to be sure that there is a common understanding of anorexia nervosa as a disorder. This requires that we spend some time considering the characteristics of anorexia -- psychological, physical, developmental, and demographic -- for which some degree of consensus can be found among mental health experts. Following this, the two most common forms of eating disorder, anorexia nervosa and bulimia, will be compared in order to shed some light on what anorexia is not. Analysis of risk for these disorders of eating will focus upon the specific risk factors that distinguish vulnerable women. The questions to be answered will concern whether these two risk patterns differ and whether the differences relate sensibly to symptoms of the full-blown disorders? This analysis will provide the first opportunity to present at-risk evidence from our research program. My purpose will be to solidify the position that anorectic risk is best understood as distinct from the risk of bulimia despite the fact that the same person may display both types of disorder in her lifetime.

Characteristics Specific to Anorexia Nervosa

The Diagnostic Manual. Description of a behavior disorder often begins with the Diagnostic and Statistical Manual published by the American Psychiatric Association (revised 3rd edition, 1987; DSM-IIIR). This popular diagnostic sourcebook lists four essential features defining anorexia nervosa. The person (1) refuses to maintain body weight beyond a minimum standard for age and height, (2) evidences an intense fear of gaining weight or becoming fat despite being underweight, (3) shows a fattened distortion of body image, and (4) ceases to menstruate.

Reduction in total food intake, often accompanied by heavy exercise, leads to weight loss in the anorectic woman, and she is likely to come to professional attention when the loss becomes marked (i.e., down to 85% of expected weight). When profoundly underweight, the person may also display a number of other abnormal physical signs -- low body temperature, a slowed heartbeat, low blood pressure, collection of body fluids, hair not unlike a new-born baby, and a variety of metabolic changes.

People receive the diagnosis of anorexia nervosa as early as in their teens and as late as the early 30s. The ratio of women to men who display anorexia is thought to be about 19 to 1. Base rate for the disorder according to the Diagnostic Manual can be as high as 1 in 100 females in the general population. However, I have seen considerably higher prevalence rates cited for populations of college women in research reports (i.e., 5-10%) and have received unofficial estimates of even higher figures within certain women's social organizations on my own campus. Seemingly, how frequently you encounter the anorectic disorder in women depends upon where you look.

Death by starvation or by breakdown in vital bodily functions represent the greatest dangers associated with anorexia, and hospitalization may be required to avoid these dire consequences. Psychological repercussions of the anorectic condition also are devastating as the person plays out a consuming obsession with food, eating, and body thinness.

Models of anorectic development. Anorexia nervosa has attracted a number of personality-based explanations that extend its distinguishing characteristics beyond the basic symptomatic and demographic features offered by DSM-IIIR (e.g., Garner, Olmstead, & Polivy, 1983; Slade, 1982). The developmental markers of anorexia nervosa, for which there is some consensus among clinical theorists, represent an important source of risk factors for our research.

Slade's (1982) developmental model for anorexia nervosa offers an interesting theoretical treatment of how adolescents progress from frustration and conflict to excessive dieting and starvation. Dieting becomes an activity of choice, since it is an insular activity that promises a degree of control and a certainty of success. These are not seen as possible within other spheres of accomplishment in which others play more critical roles. According to Slade, the adolescent may be drawn into overzealous dieting if she is made desperate by her self-perceived failure within what I have identified as the two principle domains of achievement. Whether she is realistic in her assessments or not, the adolescent suffers a crisis of self-esteem, because progress toward career success and toward interpersonal success, particularly heterosexual, appears to be floundering. Sense of achievement is diminished by unrealistic standards of perfection that come from the family and are accepted by the adolescent. Although these unrealistic standards are more explicitly tied to school achievement and career preparation by the Slade model, perfectionism can be just as detrimental within the interpersonal sphere. The adolescent who is prey to perfectionism while competing for success in school seems a likely candidate to hold unrealistic standards for interpersonal success.

Garner et al. (1983) suggest a similar set of dynamics in anoretic development as they selected the essential features of anorexia nervosa for their Eating Disorders Inventory (which was used in our program of research). The questionnaire's scale of Ineffectiveness probes the sense of failure and low self-esteem suffered by the anorectic, and Interpersonal Distrust items extend the absence of accomplishment into social relationships. Garner and his group, like Slade, emphasize the unrealistic standards of the anorectic in their Perfectionism scale.

Beside achievement failures within career-preparation and interpersonal domains, put into bold relief by perfectionism, the Slade model also emphasizes the importance of the adolescent's conflict regarding the assumption of adult roles. The same can be said for Garner and his colleagues who include a scale measuring Maturity Fears. Given the female's view of her lack of accomplishment, it is not surprising that she looks ahead to the adult years with considerable trepidation. Looking backward wistfully to the less responsible and undemanding childhood roles of years past would be an understandable preference. Two more scales complete the Garner et al. assessment of critical anorectic features. Drive for Thinness probes the basic concern with body weight, and Interoceptive Awareness considers the confusion regarding inner sensations and the feared loss of control over these feelings.

Given self-perceived failure in the two important domains of accomplishment and the low self-esteem that accompanies it, the Slade model proposes that adolescents may select an option that promises to reintroduce control in their lives and a chance at success. A thin body, highly valued in American girls at least back to age 10 (McGovern, 1988), may be achieved by dieting and exercise. Since food restraint or exercise can be pursued by the individual with little involvement of outsiders, the person is in a better position to determine progress and outcome. I would add that by abdicating standard domains of attainment and substituting self-determined success in achieving a thin body, the female reduces the importance of open competition with other people as a determinant of who succeeds and who does not. She can choose to be a "closet competitor" as she privately compares her body to those of other women or simply rely on her own personal standards of thinness. Unfortunately for the woman's wellbeing, the psychological changes that are involved in anorectic development make her a poor judge of her own success in pursuing thinness.

The four aspects of adolescent failure dynamics represented in the Slade and Garner et al. explanations of anorectic development (achievement failure, lack of interpersonal success, perfectionism, and conflict over the assumption of adult roles) will serve as an important risk indicator in our studies. These predisposing factors, along with priority given to body thinness and problems with inner sensations, make up the symptom pattern we used as one of the basic risk variables in our research. Evidence of this pattern in our subjects represented the "budding symptoms" of the disorder which, along with excesses of stress, helped us identify additional specific indicators of anorectic vulnerability in young-adult women exposed to competitive pressures for achievement.

Stress is not ignored as a dynamic factor in anorectic development by Slade and the Garner group, but it does not receive as much attention as I think it deserves as a risk variable. It is in the importance attributed to stress that my own efforts to understand the transition from frustrated achievement striving to dysfunctional eating depart from their proposals. My emphasis upon the presence of extraordinary stress levels among females who are at some greater risk of becoming anoretic makes sense to me for a number of reasons. If nothing more, high stress serves to verify the presence and importance of a pervasive sense of failure, reluctance to assume adult roles that loom perilously close ahead, and a disconcerting inner milieu for the college female. If she is bothered by her floundering development, it should be evident in the amount of stress she experiences. Since our investigations were conducted using subjects from a normal college population and not in a clinic, it became imperative that we have some basis for distinguishing between women who were seriously bothered by these developmental problems and those who were exposed to the same problems but took them more in stride. It is assumed that if the self-perceived achievement failures associated with anorexia nervosa reach significant proportions and are accompanied by serious life stress, their problem status is confirmed and the risk of anorexia seems a matter for greater concern.

High stress not only contributes to an improved research methodology by verifying the disturbing qualities of faulty development for the higher-risk women, but it also serves a theoretical purpose in my effort to place risk factors in some meaningful dynamic context. The properties of stress help explain why the woman acquires anorectic symptoms and how these symptoms are maintained. The initial motiva-

tion for achieving bodily thinness as a substitute goal is likely generated in large measure by the stress of self-perceived failure. The deci
sion to relinquish the priority given to career and interpersonal goals to
pursue her own version of success in the form of a thin body would
represent an effort to reduce this aversive motivation. Furthermore, it is
likely that the dynamics of anorectic development include stress as a
major source of motivation for food restraint long after the switch in
goal priority has been effected. Stress continues for the female at-risk
for anorexia because of her self-defeating reluctance to recognize her
own thinness so that she might allow herself a full measure of substitute
success. At the same time, selection of a substitute goal for the young-
adult woman in a college setting would not fully insulate her from the
importance of the usual forms of achievement that she despairs will
elude her. Others will be around to remind her that being thin is not
enough.

Stress, then, is of paramount importance because it serves both a
methodological and a theoretical purpose. It helps to verify problem
status for presumably at-risk subjects and contributes to a sensible
psychological explanation of anorectic development by providing a
motivational dynamic. It should come as no surprise that stress will
attract more focused consideration as a basic risk factor in the next two
chapters on anorectic vulnerability.

Distinguishing Anorectic Risk from the Risk of Bulimia

To this point I have offered a description of anorexia nervosa as a
psychobiological disorder in terms of its defining symptoms and the
personality factors that antecede them for which there is some consensus among experts. There is a problem, however, in the case of
anorexia in trying to portray the disorder exclusively in terms of common characteristics. It also is important to understand anorexia nervosa
in terms of what it is not -- how it differs from bulimia. We can begin
by examining the actual properties of the bulimic disorder, but the more
critical effort to distinguish these two types of eating problems will
involve research into their respective risk indicators.

The distinction between anorexia nervosa and bulimia is blurred by
the fact that both eating disorders may appear in the clinical history of
the same individual. However, DSM-IIIR presents them as independent
disorders. Bulimia as an eating disorder begins with the person's over-
concern regarding the ingestion of food and body fatness. Despite these
concerns, the person will lapse into eating binges during which an

amazing quantity of food is eaten, usually in private. After a lengthy session of binge eating, the bulimic will engage in some form of purging in which the person evacuates the food she has eaten by means of purgatives or, commonly, by induced vomiting. Bulimia is found in almost 5% of college women, nine times more frequently than for their male peers.

A strategy of weight control can be noted in symptomatic behaviors of the bulimic just as was evident in the symptoms of anorexia nervosa. Both types of disorder involve some means of curtailing weight gain about which they are so preoccupied. The bulimic uses purging to prevent weight gain in the wake of her eating sprees. The anorectic loses weight or maintains skeletal thinness by restricting her food intake. One promising way to distinguish between the two disorders as ultimate risks is to focus upon these strategies of weight control and try to answer complementary questions. Why do some weight-conscious women lapse into eating binges, which force them to purge their excesses, rather than simply maintaining a restrictive diet? Examining the other side of the same coin, the question becomes why other women, also concerned about body weight, are capable of maintaining a diet and unlikely to submit to binge eating?

The empirical evidence to be presented rests on the observation that dieting is a commonplace and effective method of losing weight among females and that purging is an improvised procedure required by dysfunctional eating binges in the weight-conscious woman. Dieting should be the preferred strategy for the woman concerned about weight control unless her efforts to restrict food intake have proven unsuccessful. Cognitive liabilities hampering self-control would work against eating restraint and favor a bulimic solution in two ways. They would make it more difficult to resist the temptation to eat when hungry, and they would make uncontrolled binge eating more likely. In short, a deficit in self-control should reduce the risk of anorexia nervosa that would require self-restraint with regard to food and increase bulimic risk involving unrestrained eating in weight-conscious women. At a given point in time, then, the risk of bulimia is incompatible with the risk of anorexia to the extent that cognitive limitations disallow effective food restraint. That both disorders have been noted in the clinical history of the same weight-conscious woman would have to be explained in part by changes in the psychological conditions governing the effectiveness of dieting, self-control among them.

Poor self-control as an explanation for dieting failure and binge eating. To repeat the premise emphasized above, reducing weight requires self-control if it is to be successful. Hunger is highly motivating and food is usually accessible. If the woman is not up to satisfying the restrictions of dieting, she will not achieve or sustain the weight loss required to meet her own goals. Those who lack the self-control to diet successfully can be just as concerned about their weight as successful dieters but must work around their deficits in self-regulation to deal with these concerns in other ways. If poor self-control compromises efforts at sustained dieting and, worse, if this poor self-restraint sets the stage for rampages of eating, a bulimic outcome may be at-risk. She deals with her uncontrolled eating episodes in the best way she can so that they at least will not add to her girth; purging, usually by self-induced vomiting, removes the food.

Heilbrun and Bloomfield (1986) considered the role of self-control in bulimic risk using a sample of 57 college females. The strategy of research in which questionnaire information obtained from the subject is used to identify symptomatic beginnings was used; this procedure already has been described in general terms for probing the risk of anorexia. The two scales from the Eating Disorders Inventory (EDI; Garner, Olmstead, & Polivy, 1983) that deal with bulimic characteristics were combined into a single score, after converting their raw scores to a common standard score to equalize their importance. This "bulimic profile" (BP) was considered a general index of risk for a bulimic disorder as it involved the admission of bulimic characteristics at some level. The two scales included Bulimia, which contains items inquiring into binge eating and purging, and Body Dissatisfaction, a compilation of items bearing upon perceived fatness of and displeasure with certain body parts.

Self-control was approached conceptually as a multidimensional capability in which self-regulation depends upon a number of cognitive skills or styles. The conclusion that self-control can be usefully conceptualized in multidimensional cognitive terms evolved from an early investigation of addicted male and female alcoholics and their controls (Heilbrun, Tarbox, & Madison, 1979). Alcoholics offered an ideal population for investigating a deficit in self-regulation, since they not only lack the ability to control their drinking in particular, but by case description show poorly controlled, irresponsible behaviors in general. The 1979 investigation and other studies of self-control deficits in alcoholism (Heilbrun & Abraham, 1987; Heilbrun, Cassidy, Diehl, Haas, & Heilbrun, 1986; Heilbrun & Norbert, 1972; Heilbrun &

Schwartz, 1980) revealed that self-control is multifaceted, governed by a number of cognitive functions that operate independently of each other. Three functions were identified. Each represented an important source of self-control problems in the alcoholic with prominence depending upon the stage of alcoholism (Heilbrun & Abraham, 1987). Even though these studies of self-control deficit concentrated upon adult diagnosed alcoholics under treatment, the implications carry over to juvenile offenders and even into a college population like that sampled by Heilbrun and Bloomfield. The three self-control factors and the laboratory tasks used to measure them were found to be equally effective in revealing deficits of self-regulation within samples of problem drinkers made up from juvenile court cases and students on a college campus (Heilbrun, Cassidy, Diehl, Haas, & Heilbrun, 1986).

The three cognitive sources of self-control (in no special order) include the ability to restrain acting on impulse through self-instruction (impulse control). Perhaps this basis for self-regulation most readily comes to mind when self-control is considered. A second source of self-control involves the person's sensitivity to and utilization of internal cues as information relevant to taking action (reflectiveness or internal scanning). Reflectiveness, probably less familiar as a source of self-control, involves consideration of relevant information before choosing to act. Review could include symbolic information that is derived from recalling past experience, weighing values, or utilizing reasoning and judgment. Reflection as a source of self-control also would cover the person's sensitivity to body sensations relevant to an action. Taking another drink when inebriated (for alcoholics) and eating more despite being full (for bulimics) are examples of insensitivity to internal stimulation contributing to poor self-control. The third source of self-control that has been studied is self-reinforcement, the person's ability to influence her future action through self-evaluation of past conduct. Your own disapproval or approval of a particular action should inhibit or promote that behavior if you are capable of effective self-reinforcement.

The four laboratory tasks used in the Heilbrun and Bloomfield (1986) study to measure self-control factors in bulimic risk were selected from the battery used in the series of investigations involving alcoholics and problem drinkers that have been cited previously. They will not be described in detail here. Those interested in the specific procedures are encouraged to consult the 1986 Heilbrun and Abraham paper. There are a few general comments about the original self-control battery that deserve mention, however. The nature of these self-control tasks was such as to allow administration without calling attention to what was being measured. Subtlety of instruction and task was intended to avoid cognitive performance that was out of character for the subject because of unique experimental demands. Another point has to do with the correlations between scores on the tasks. There may be concern that the three self-control functions seriously overlap one another, particularly impulsiveness and reflection as opposite sides of the same coin. Distinct contributions by the three self-control factors is assured by their factor-analytic origins in which independence is required and by the fact that subsequent studies have found them to be uncorrelated with each other.

Returning to the study of bulimic risk and self-control, error scores for the four self-control tasks were converted into standard score distributions with a mean of 50 and a standard deviation of 10. The tasks included two measuring impulse control and two involving reflective cognition; the self-reinforcement task was not included because of time constraints. The research question concerned whether college women at-risk for bulimia (high BP) had poorer self-control than women for whom bulimia is an unlikely prospect. The median or mid-point on the combined scores for the Bulimia and Body Dissatisfaction scales was used to split the female sample into BP levels. The average impulsiveness error score for high BP women ($\underline{M}$ = 51.68) was above that found for low BP (49.02), and the difference proved to be significant ($\underline{p}$ < .05). The comparison for reflectiveness, scored inversely, provided the same result. High BP subjects considered internally-generated information less ($\underline{M}$ = 52.23) than did controls ($\underline{M}$ = 48.31, $\underline{p}$ < .05). The research question was answered in the affirmative; women identified by the EDI as at some greater risk for bulimia were inferior to controls in two cognitive functions crucial to self-control.

While risk of a bulimic disorder and binge eating, its predominant symptom, were found to be associated with limited self-control in college women, an equally crucial question follows this demonstration. It is still necessary to show that women at anorectic risk can be distinguished from high BP women in level of self-control. To contend with this question, Heilbrun and Bloomfield examined the relationship between risk and self-control after reshuffling their sample into high and low anorectic-profile (AP) subjects. This reanalysis was based upon a median-split of the remaining six EDI scales after their raw scores were transformed to a common standard scale and combined. If

the risk of anorexia nervosa and of bulimia are to be considered independent at a particular point in time, the same deficits in self-control
should not be apparent when high AP women are compared to their
controls. This is difficult to demonstrate using our questionnaire
approach to identifying basic risk groups, since the AP and BP scores
are correlated with each other ($\underline{r}$ in the .50s over different samples).
What is found for one risk group will tend to show up for the other.
This overlap is not surprising when you consider that any weight-
conscious woman is likely to score high on both the Body Dissatisfaction scale heralding bulimic risk and Drive for Thinness scale indicating anorectic risk.

When the two self-control deficit scores were examined for AP
groups, there was no hint of self-control differences. Impulse-control
error scores for the high AP women ($\underline{M}$ = 50.61) and their controls ($\underline{M}$
= 50.12) were very similar. The same result was obtained when high
AP ($\underline{M}$ =49.50) and low AP ($\underline{M}$ = 50.24) females were compared on
reflectiveness; women at anorectic risk were slightly more reflective
than their controls though not significantly so statistically. The conclusion suggested by the parallel BP and AP analyses is that the self-
control required for food restraint is more likely to be represented in
women generally at-risk for anorexia, whereas deficits in self-control in
the form of impulsive and unreflective behavior that would contribute
to failed dieting and binge eating are more characteristic of women who
appear vulnerable to a bulimic disorder.

One further analysis would be in order for those who might call for
a more direct comparison in self-control for college females at-risk for
bulimia and others at anorectic risk according to the EDI. Ten women
in the sample fell above the sample mid-point on the BP score and
below the mid-point on the AP score; by my research definition, these
women are at-risk for bulimia (but not anorexia). Nine subjects showed
the opposite pattern and can be considered at anorectic risk (but not
bulimic risk). These small groups were directly compared on self-
control after combining all individual reflectiveness and impulsivity
scores into a single composite index. I did this to increase score
reliability in anticipation of a comparison between very small groups.
Reflectiveness scores were reversed in meaning, so that high scores
conveyed a lower degree of reflection. High index scores, then, suggested poor self-control in terms of unreflective and impulsive action.

Direct comparison found women at-risk for bulimic problems with
an average self-control score of 208.20 and the anorectic-risk group

with an average composite index of 191.89. The difference was significant statistically ($\underline{p}$ < .01). Also important, absolute values of these
means mark the bulimic-risk group as clearly below average in self-
control and the anorectic-risk group just as evidently above average
relative to the mean index score for the entire sample of college women
($\underline{M}$ = 201.61).

Insensitivity to satiety cues as a risk factor in bulimia. Problems in
self-control are a valuable way of explaining less success at food
restraint when overweight is a concern for the college woman at-risk for
bulimia. They also do double duty by explaining the occasional lapse
into binges of overeating. The eating excesses of binging are so
dramatic, however, they seem to require additional explanation. What
other trait might logically explain massive food intake within a
restricted time-frame for a weight-conscious female? Perhaps the most
obvious candidate would be some aspect of cognition that would limit
her ability to respond to satiety cues signaling fullness. The internal
sensations associated with satiety encourage us to terminate eating, and
this warning system seems singularly lacking in binge eating when food
intake continues beyond normal and even further beyond the proscriptions of diet. We are told that sensations marking satiety work independently of hunger level in the regulation of food intake (Kissileff,
Thornton, & Becker, 1982; Smith & Gibbs, 1979; Teghtsoonian, Becker, & Edelman, 1981). It remains possible, then, that binge eaters continue to eat not because they remain hungry but because they fail to
respond to the sensations of satiety.

We approached this next investigation not only with the idea that a
collaboration of cognitive deficits would be likely if the excesses of
binge eating are to be understood but with the anticipation that a more
formidable distinction could be made between anorectic and bulimic
risk. The weight-conscious woman at-risk for bulimia might succumb
to hunger because she lacked self-control, and the same problem with
self-control would make it difficult to keep the quantity of food
ingested within reasonable limits when she did. It would require some
degree of failure in the "turn-off" mechanism provided by satiety cues
to enhance the chances of continuing the intake of food to the
extraordinary lengths found in bulimic binges, however. Neither type
of cognitive deficit should be found in women at anorectic risk.

Heilbrun and Worobow (1991) considered whether college females
at-risk for bulimia lacked responsiveness to satiety cues and whether
this deficit, if found, set them apart from females exposed to the risk of

anorexia nervosa. A rating-scale approach to studying responsiveness was employed; there was no logistically feasible alternative for examining the very private and inaccessible sensations of satiety. The first 5-point rating scale inquired into <u>awareness</u>, the degree to which the woman was typically aware of sensations indicating she had eaten enough during a routine meal. The second 5-point scale considered <u>imperative</u> action; how readily does the woman stop eating when she does become aware of being full? Comparable scales also were presented to the subjects in which "drinking" was substituted for "eating" in considering the two aspects of responsiveness. These control ratings were used to examine whether any results obtained with regard to eating satiety cues would generalize to drinking satiety effects. In other words, is insensitivity to food satiety sensations part of a more general deficit in attention?

We were concerned that our self-ratings of responsiveness to satiety cues would not be powerful enough to disclose the deficits under investigation even if they existed, so we attempted to refine our measurement procedures by considering another facet of attention that might contribute to these effects. The extent to which any pattern of stimulation reaches our awareness or compels some responsive action depends in part upon how effectively the person is deploying her attention at the time. If she is distracted or is otherwise not concentrating well, sensations are more likely to be inaccurately received or to be missed altogether. The poorer the reception, the less imperative the message.

The relevance of this observation to the Heilbrun and Worobow methodology is that there are differences between individuals in how they <u>routinely</u> deploy attention to stimulation (Nideffer, 1973). These attentional styles include the particular parameter of attention in which we were especially interested -- the effectiveness of attention when it is committed to stimulation. Some are simply not as good at focusing their attention as others. If a woman were generally less capable of focusing her attention or maintaining a focus, her responsiveness to satiety cues would be expected to suffer along with her response to other sensations. The methodological implication here is that effectiveness of attentional focus should be considered along with the BP score in order to establish whether cues of satiety tend to be lost as part of the bulimic risk picture. The prediction would be that a deficit in response to eating satiety would be found in a subset of high BP college women who are generally less capable of narrowing their focus of attention in an effective way. Maintaining the distinction between women at-risk for anorexia and for bulimia would require that this complex result be obtained for high BP subjects and not for high AP subjects.

Nideffer's (1973) Test of Attentional and Interpersonal Styles (TAIS) was employed as a measure of attention deployment. The self-report items disclose individual differences in the way people attend to stimulation, the quality of their attention, as well as differences in the intensity of stimulation to which people are exposed. Six scales of attentional styles and the conditions that command attention are scored, but only one TAIS scale was subjected to analysis in the Heilbrun and Worobow study. This 13-item Narrow Effective Focus (NAR) scale depicts an individual able to concentrate by narrowing attention at the high end to someone whose focused attention is disrupted by irrelevant stimuli at the low end. As an example, studying involves a narrowing of attention to whatever is being studied. Some individuals are more capable than others in attending to the object of study and shutting out irrelevant and potentially distracting stimulation. A second example brings us back to the subject at hand. Some people are better able to attend to satiety cues and not be distracted by other stimulation that is competing for attention.

The average awareness and imperative action ratings for sensations of hunger satiety are found in Table 3.1. Median score values for the entire sample of 80 college women were used to define high and low BP females and to further subdivide the BP groups into high and low ability to narrow attention effectively. Statistical evaluation of the awareness score revealed only one overall effect, an interaction ($p < .01$). This can be explained by the distinctly low awareness of hunger satiety cues in high BP women who report some general problem in narrowing their attention ($M = 2.88$) that contrasts with other high BP women more capable of focusing attention ($M = 3.88$, $p < .005$). The same effect was not observed in low BP women for whom poorer and better attentional focus had no apparent influence upon the awareness of hunger satiety cues. Only women at bulimic risk who also have a general problem focusing their attention report limited awareness of satiety cues.

Ratings of the action taken by the woman in response to satiety cues revealed the same pattern of results. A strong interaction ($p < .001$) emerged when high BP subjects with problems in attentional focusing rated themselves as less compelled by satiety cues ($M = 2.56$) than other high BP subjects more capable of focusing ($M = 3.44$), $p < .001$. This difference did not show up when low BP subjects were broken down by

Table 3.1.   Sensitivity to Hunger Satiety Cues Among College Women Ordered by Bulimic and Anorectic Characteristics and by Effective Focusing of Attention

	Awareness of Satiety Cues $\underline{M}$	Imperative Action Groups $\underline{M}$
High BP		
Effective Focus ($\underline{N}$ = 16)	3.88	3.44
Ineffective Focus ($\underline{N}$ = 25)	2.88	2.56
Low BP		
Effective Focus ($\underline{N}$ = 23)	3.39	3.09
Ineffective Focus ($\underline{N}$ = 16)	3.62	3.50
High AP		
Effective Focus ($\underline{N}$ = 18)	3.33	3.00
Ineffective Focus ($\underline{N}$ = 21)	3.43	3.33
Low AP		
Effective Focus ($\underline{N}$ = 21)	3.48	3.33
Ineffective Focus ($\underline{N}$ = 20)	3.55	3.30

Note. - Taken in part from Heilbrun, A.B., & Worobow, A. L. (1991). Attention and disordered eating behavior: I. Disattention to satiety cues as a risk factor in development of bulimia. Journal of Clinical Psychology, 47, 3-9.

effectiveness of focus. Only high BP and low NAR females report a clearcut deficit in acting upon sensations of satiety when they do register.

Both sets of results clearly suggest that the failure to respond to hunger satiety cues appears only in one subset of college women who qualify as being at bulimic risk. Women who endorse bulimic symptoms and who are generally prone to problems in focusing attention on specific stimuli also report an insensitivity to sensations that normally deter further eating. They also tend to ignore these warning signs to the extent they do register. Both make binging behavior more understandable.

The parallel analyses of the awareness and imperative action scores, after regrouping subjects by high and low AP and further subdividing them by high and low NAR (see lower half of Table 3.1), revealed no semblance of a relationship. This result (unreported in the journal article), like that found in the study of self-control, is particularly striking in light of the fact that the regrouping was accomplished by using a risk score that was positively correlated with the BP metric. There were no differences in responsiveness to satiety cues for the AP groupings despite the correlation.

The examination of thirst satiety sensations revealed much the same pattern as was found for hunger satiety. High BP, low NAR women reported less awareness ($\underline{M}$ = 2.92) and assigned a less imperative character ($\underline{M}$ = 2.76) in describing sensations of thirst satiety than did high BP women with a generally more effective focus of attention ($\underline{M}$ = 3.62 and 3.31, respectively, $\underline{ps}$ < .05). No trends were evident in the low BP group or in either the high or low AP groups. It would appear that there is a generalized lack of responsiveness to satiety cues in women at-risk for bulimia if they are otherwise limited in ability to focus their attention upon focal stimulation.

It has been demonstrated that bulimic risk and anorectic risk can be distinguished empirically despite the correlation between risk measures. Furthermore, both the self-control and hunger satiety results offer sensible explanations for the bulimic's failure in dieting and lapses into binge eating. The factors explaining bulimic risk do not qualify empirically or conceptually as signs of vulnerability to an anorectic disorder. These distinguishing preclinical features provide a basis for understanding women at anorectic risk not only in terms of the presence of shared attributes but also in terms of differences from women at bulimic risk.

Personality Factors and General Predisposition to Anorectic Risk

Earlier in the book I proposed a link between the young-adult woman's sense of failure in competing for career and social goals and anorectic risk. It was suggested that the failure to see herself progressing toward a successful career or marriage was in some measure fostered by perfectionistic standards and by a perceived conflict between the two goals. Other considerations no doubt add to her pessimism, including the realities of academic career preparation and social ambition that may limit opportunity to achieve no matter how tenacious the woman may be. Since the usual forms of goal attainment appear out of reach and her prospects for successful adult roles are dim, the proposal continues, a more immediate substitute goal under better personal control assumes priority. A thin body, to be gained by food restriction primarily, represents an achievement having almost universal appeal to women in western societies.

The research of interest in this chapter sought the risk factors that promised to predict which college women would reach this choicepoint and then choose the substitute goal of body thinness. In a real sense, the remaining studies of anorectic risk, to be described in the next two chapters, will address the question of why their pursuit of a thin body is so successful that they starve themselves into skeletal proportions.

The elucidation of risk factors that may serve as a general predisposition to an anorectic progression actually has begun with the studies that identified factors of importance in distinguishing between anorectic and bulimic risk, especially bulimic binge eating. Bulimic risk seems to involve poorer self-control and an attention deficit. Women concerned about body size, but who neither lack self-control nor experience a deficit in focused attention that would blur sensations of satiety, are unlikely candidates for bulimia at a given point in their lives.

Having considered anorectic risk by what it is not, I will now consider several personality variables that would help explain why some women reach the point where the dangerous shift in goal priority occurs. These questions will attract our attention. Why is the competitive element of goal-seeking not more successful? Why are the problems of perceived failure not confronted more constructively before standard achievement goals are relinquished? Why does the at-risk woman choose to switch her investment of ambition into achieving a thin body? Answers to these questions concerning failed competitive effort, poor problem resolution, and body priority will set the stage for the next chapter. There I will begin developing a picture of how stress not only signals the risk of symptom development and a full-blown anorectic disorder but escalates the danger.

Why do some females reach the point where they face seemingly insurmountable achievement problems due in large measure to their inability to compete? If you think about it, the attainment of career and interpersonal goals as an adult about exhausts the constructive possibilities when it comes to satisfying a motive to succeed (or not to fail) in our society. Since I view competition as an essential feature of success-striving within both domains, it follows that those who are reluctant to compete or who otherwise do not handle competition well will more likely have achievement problems. If you are not motivated toward success, of course, whether you are equipped to compete or not is less important. Women within our largely middle-class college samples understand the need to compete in order to stay in the hunt for society's tokens of success, although they might not be psychologically prepared to do it.

Who within a female college population would most likely be penalized by a reluctance or inability to compete? One prime candidate is the female who has adopted the traditional feminine sex-role for women in western societies. The essence of the feminine role, as popularly conceived by sex-role researchers, is an expressive orientation -- the concern with harmonious relationships between people, especially between the expressive person and others. By giving rewards the expressive role player hopes to receive rewards (Parsons & Bales, 1955). Interpersonal harmony and mutually-rewarding transactions are inimical to effective competitive effort. Qualities such as warmth, sympathy, cooperativeness, and sensitivity are mainstays of expressive transaction. None of these feminine qualities lends itself to being competitive; in fact, they all limit competitiveness.

On the other hand, the essence of the traditional male role, an instrumental orientation, is more than compatible with competitive behavior. This orientation requires that individuals maintain a personal goal-directedness, no matter what the situation, and that they be able to disregard the hostility generated by such obvious interest in self-enhancement (Parsons & Bales, 1955). Although an instrumental orientation can show itself outside the competitive arena, it is, nonetheless, a formidable basis for competing. Being concerned only about achieving your own goals and being oblivious to how people react to you would certainly facilitate competitive performance. Two studies from our program considered feminine and masculine sex-role identity in college females in order to establish whether sex-role can serve as anorectic risk indicator and to indirectly cast light on their relationship to competition and achievement problems.

Heilbrun and Mulqueen (1987) reported several bodies of data in which sex-roles were compared regarding their adaptive value in college females. One of the studies reported in the Heilbrun and Mulqueen paper considered masculine and feminine sex-role dispositions as they might relate to the risk of anorexia nervosa. Risk was gauged by the anorectic profile (AP), the sum of the six anorectic scales from the EDI.

The sex-roles considered in the Heilbrun and Mulqueen study were measured by a self-report technique that required the subject to rate the relevance of a number of masculine and feminine traits in describing her characteristic behavior in each of several different interpersonal situations. Rated behaviors emphasized the importance of feminine traits in some situations and masculine traits in others, as was expected. Scoring rules were developed by which these ratings defined the woman as primarily feminine or primarily masculine within any given situation by the priority given to sex-typed alternatives in describing her typical behavior. The woman's overall gender-role commitment was determined by a different set of rules and based on a count across the array of situations. Given that competition would be more difficult for traditional females, primarily feminine women should be more vulnerable to failures in achievement and a more serious anorectic risk within my scheme of things. On the other hand, competition would be fully compatible with masculinity. This should reduce the chance of achievement failure and diminish anorectic risk; AP scores should be lower in primarily masculine college women.

The results confirmed these expectations. The 10 primarily feminine subjects obtained higher AP scores ($\underline{M}$ = 22.70), whereas the 11 primarily masculine women were low on these scores ($\underline{M}$ = 12.63). This difference in anorectic risk was significant ($\underline{p}$ < .05). These results, taken literally, tell us that feminine college women report more of the achievement and maturity problems central to the development of anorexia than do masculine college women. My further conclusion is that this difference results in some measure from the personality traits associated with each sex-role that inhibit (femininity) or facilitate (masculinity) competitive behavior. This will be clearly supported by evidence reported later in the book when more competitive college women were found to be on the masculine side and less competitive women to be more feminine (Heilbrun, Wydra & Friedberg, 1989).

Sex-role commitment can be investigated in a number of ways. One approach would be in terms of the kind of behaviors displayed by the subject and the degree to which these behaviors corresponded to social stereotypes of masculinity and femininity. The Heilbrun and Mulqueen (1987) study that was just discussed followed that procedure. Another approach would be to examine sex-role commitment in terms of cognitive sensitivity; how attuned is the person to traditional differences between the sex-roles? A second minor wave of sex-role research has considered "gender schemas" as just such a sensitivity variable. Research experience has taught me that a different portrayal of sex-role commitment can emerge if manifest sex-role behavior and cognitive gender-schema measures are obtained from the same individual. Role commitment may vary depending upon whether private thought or public behavior is being considered.

The term "gender schema" sounds more formidable than is really the case. Schemas in general are viewed as cognitive networks (mental associations) that include information relating to some common theme. People maintain a schema including information relating to animals, for example, that would include everything the individual relates to this concept. The person's response to some stimulus that fits into an existing schema is influenced by how well developed that schema may be for the particular individual.

How does the organized body of information, attitudes, and values making up a schematic network affect how exposure to a relevant stimulus will be experienced by the person? A well-developed schema will help insure that the stimulus is noticed in the first place, that it will be given meaning in line with the schema, and that it will be remembered. For example, someone interested and well-versed in plant life is more likely to notice a small flower on a stroll, assign it some meaning within her plant schema, and remember the encounter later on.

The gender schema includes information concerning traditional sex-role stereotypes and guides the person's expectations for women and men in a given culture (Bem, 1981a). If the gender schema is strong, the person will see the world in terms of traditional distinctions between men and women. Given a weak gender schema, stereotyped role assignments will have only limited influence upon the woman's behavior or experience. Whether she turns out to be feminine or masculine (or both), she does so with little regard for what has previously distinguished women and men.

Heilbrun and Putter (1986) compared strength of the gender schema in college females at-risk for anorexia and their controls. Before presenting these results, a word about measurement procedures for this cognitive variable would be in order. Generally speaking, the measurement of gender schema as a mental organization is more complicated than the measurement of manifest sex-role behaviors, since subjects would be expected to report more readily about their public behaviors than they can about their mental organizations. One solution to this measurement dilemma is to concentrate on what people do that would be related to the strength of a gender schema and not on their observations about how their minds function. This assumes, of course, that a switch from probing private introspection to examining public behavior is possible for the researcher.

The consensus among gender-schema researchers is that what an individual does in way of memory for stereotyped sex-role information represents a readily-measured indicator of schema strength (Bem, 1981a; Heilbrun, 1986; Madison, 1983; Mills, 1983). Expose a person to some piece of information relevant to traditional roles for men and women without any special instructions to remember what has been seen or heard. Theoretically, such stereotypic information is more likely to be selected out and remembered if the information fits into a well-developed gender schema. Turn this theoretical given around, and you have a basis for measuring an unobserved mental organization. If your subjects remember stereotypic information better, they possess more fully developed gender schemas.

Heilbrun and Putter used a laboratory procedure to measure gender schema in which 69 college women were visually presented sex-typed information embedded in a larger number of non-sex-typed items. The subjects were asked to remember as much of the information (stereotyped and nonstereotyped personality traits) as they could following presentation, although no distinction was made between the two types of traits. The extent to which sex-typed items were selectively remembered was used to gauge strength of gender schema. The EDI was used, as always, to develop an anorectic-profile score for estimating risk.

At first blush, results of the Heilbrun and Putter study of gender schemas appear to contradict those of Heilbrun and Mulqueen (1987) reported earlier which considered manifest sex-role behaviors. The 1987 evidence suggested that college females who were traditionally feminine in their self-reported sex-role behaviors demonstrated greater anorectic risk than nontraditional masculine females. Analysis of gender schemas, the female's sensitivity to traditional sex-role stereotypes, revealed just the opposite effect. Using the median AP score as the dividing point, the 34 high AP women obtained an average gender-schema score of 33.08 compared to an average score of 43.03 for the 35 low AP women. Greater vulnerability to anorexia was associated with less sensitivity to traditional masculine and feminine expectations relative to controls ($p < .05$). The apparent contradiction resides in the opposite-direction findings that women at-risk were shown to be less traditional by gender-schema measurement and more traditional by a sex-role behavior measure.

What appears to be a gross contradiction in the relationship between traditional sex-role commitment and risk for anorexia was resolvable, quite fortunately, because stress level had been included as an additional risk factor in the Heilbrun and Putter gender-schema study. The availability of a stress measure in this preliminary study allowed us to discover an effect that would have otherwise remained masked by our initial findings. Table 3.2 presents the level of daily stress reported by the women in the Heilbrun and Putter study after they are broken down by both anorectic risk and strength of gender schema. (How stress was measured will be covered in the next chapter.)

As Table 3.2 clearly portrays, high AP females with a stronger gender schema reported singularly elevated stress, significantly ($p < .05$) above the level of any other group. Reading the three-way relationships a different way, women at the greatest risk for anorectic development (high AP scores and under high stress) revealed stronger gender schemas. Both the Heilbrun and Mulqueen and the Heilbrun and Putter studies, then, point to the same conclusion. A commitment to the traditional role for women, either in terms of sex-role behavior or a greater sensitivity to traditional sex-role distinctions between women and men, puts the college female at higher risk for anorexia. The expressive orientation, at the heart of traditional femininity, looms as a major problem for the at-risk college woman as it interferes with competitiveness in a situation where competition is essential. Stifled competitiveness, in turn, helps explain the faltering attainment of the woman at-risk for anorexia.

Why are the problems of perceived failure not more constructively confronted before standard achievement goals are relinquished? If feminine behavior and sensitivity to traditional feminine expectations con tribute to stressful problems in competition and attainment for at-risk

Table 3.2. Stress Level for College Females at More and Less Anorectic Risk and with Stronger and Weaker Gender Schemas

	More Anorectic Risk (High AP)		Less Anorectic Risk (Low AP)	
Gender Schema	N	M	N	M
Stronger	14	54.71	22	36.45
Weaker	20	44.30	13	42.23

Note. - Adapted from Heilbrun, A. B., & Putter, L. D. (1986). Preoccupation with stereotyped sex-role differences, ideal body weight, and stress in college women showing anorexic characteristics. International Journal of Eating Disorders, 5, 1035-1049.

women, it remains to be seen why these women do not do a more effective job of confronting their problems and bringing stress down to more tolerable limits. My proposal regarding competitive failure as an antecedent to anorectic choice would be bolstered by an explanation for the poor problem-solving that precedes relinquishing standard goals and selecting a thin body as a compensatory achievement. My emerging interest in the role of stress in the risk of psychobiological disorder during the mid-1980s suggested one possible answer. Some college women may be slow to resolve problems because of the way they cope with stress and its sources. Perhaps the coping styles that are routinely employed when problem-based stress arises contribute in differing degree to poor problem resolution and the continuation of stress.

There are only two general approaches to relieving a stress state, although these may take myriad forms. The individual may attempt to deal directly with the source of stress, but sometimes this is not possible. The source of stress may be unknown or otherwise unmodifiable, the means of changing the stressor may not be available, or confronting the source may be risky. No matter what the exceptions may be, however, the principle remains the same -- dealing with stress at its problematic source should have coping priority. Direct action stands a chance of diminishing the effects of a stressor or removing the problem altogether.

Since direct action toward a source of stress is sometimes not an option, people tend to rely on indirect coping strategies that are far more accessible though less effective in the long run. Indirect strategies are not intended to change the problem creating stress; rather they are intended to reduce the unpleasant emotional component of stress, the "gut-wrenching" feelings that are so familiar to the stressed individual. Indirect coping is valuable to the extent that it allows for at least temporary escape from the emotional burden of stress.

Indirect coping strategies may take a variety of forms, including some that are more dangerous than others. For example, exercise activities may serve a stress-reduction function and also provide other health-related benefits. A few turns around the track, an aerobics class, or a game of tennis, and the tensions of the day may subside. Physical exercise is also inherently beneficial. At the other health extreme, alcohol consumption or other drug use can have a comparable tranquilizing effect, but the risk of misbehavior, addiction, and psychobiological damage enters the picture. Certainly the most accessible and heavily utilized procedure for dealing with stress indirectly are the various defensive styles. These involve different strategies that people employ for dealing with distressing information. Each strategy represents a different way of altering information so that it is less threatening and less capable of arousing the emotions of stress at a particular point in time. It was within the domain of the psychological defenses that we came to look for sources of problem-solving limitations in women at-risk for anorexia. To understand why the defenses came to attract our attention requires a brief review of the evidence and theory regarding these self-protective mechanisms that were available by 1986.

The number of defenses is a matter of opinion. Different theorists offer varied catalogues of the ways people protect themselves mentally from threat. Despite this diversity, there is core agreement regarding a few defenses that seem important to almost everyone and top most of the lists. These tend to derive from Freud's early works in which he formulated the role played by the defenses in mental disorders (e.g., Freud, 1911; 1915; 1938), although the core defenses do not necessarily retain his psychoanalytic assumptions. Among the major defenses bearing a Freudian stamp are repression, projection, rationalization, and denial. Despite agreement that these defenses are commonly employed to defuse unpleasant information, there is disagreement regarding their exact definition, measurement, and how they actually function.

My own approach to understanding the defenses and measuring them by laboratory procedures is made evident in a series of published studies (Heilbrun, 1972; Heilbrun, 1977; Heilbrun, 1978; Heilbrun, 1982; Heilbrun, 1984; Heilbrun, Blum, & Goldreyer, 1985; Heilbrun, Diller, & Dodson, 1986; Heilbrun & Pepe, 1985; Heilbrun & Schwartz, 1979). I have tried to reconceptualize the major defensive strategies so that they would more reasonably describe the behavior of normal individuals and psychiatric patients alike. The following represent my versions of the four major defenses.

Repression is understood to mean the selective failure to remember distressing information. The motivated memory loss, in which the person literally puts something "out of mind," need not be profound. Given the right cue, the information will usually return to awareness. However, repression can range in strength from temporarily forgetting distressing information (sometimes called "suppression") to an inability to remember that is tantamount to permanent loss. In any case, repression prevents the person from being aware of a problem that would otherwise be the source of stress.

Projection, as I use it, is a defensive operation used by people who depend upon social comparison for self-evaluation. That is, they judge their own qualities by using other people as standards. Projection occurs when people unfavorably distort the qualities of people in their social environment so that by comparison they can deny some undesirable attribute in themselves. Perceptual distortion may be of a less or more serious variety. It may involve the arbitrary selection of a particular social model whose unfavorable traits make the projector's traits seem more acceptable by comparison. In more serious cases of distortion, the person may fabricate some undesirable characteristic in a social model as a basis for favorable comparison and denial of the same characteristic in herself. This more serious distortion comes closest to "attributive projection" in psychiatric textbooks.

An example of projection, as I use the term, might be in order. If one is faced with hostility as an unacceptable personal trait, isolating a very hostile person for purposes of comparison would exemplify the less serious form of projection. Misrepresenting another person as being very hostile for sake of social comparison would represent a more serious form of projection as it involves a greater distortion of reality. Projection as illustrated here can backfire to the extent that the hostility emphasized by these perceptual tactics, especially fabrication, is believed directed toward the projector. This could encourage further distortions of thought as the projector seeks meaning and resolution to a dilemma of her own creation.

The threat that is involved in a projective defense is the recognition of something in yourself that is unacceptable. The temporary resolution of threat and reduction of stress by projection involves altering the information by convenient social comparisons. Poor problem resolution could result from the failure to confront whatever is unacceptable in oneself or from the unrealistic distortions that are introduced into one's social environment.

Rationalization involves the alteration of information so that it becomes more desirable and, therefore, less threatening. This often involves the assignment of a more acceptable motive to behaviors that would otherwise be unacceptable. When used as a defense in examining your own personality characteristics, it also includes increasing the value assigned to a personal attribute to make it more acceptable or denigrating the value of a trait if it is missing. Rationalization in this sense would soften the person's view of herself and reduce the discomfort of self-dissatisfaction. It would deter problem resolution to the extent that negative self-appraisal represents a motive for change.

Denial is the outright rejection of a piece of information without a sufficient subjective basis for doing so. Parents may be unwilling to accept an unfavorable assertion about their child even though they have no justification for assuming the assertion is false. The problem created for problem resolution is obvious; if something is denied, there is no problem. In summary, then, distress from unwelcome information may be temporarily diminished or avoided by forgetting the information, diminishing its negative impact by convenient or fabricated comparison, altering it, or denying it outright. All of these strategies could result in procrastination or worse in confronting stressful problems.

What has this discussion of indirect coping strategies, defensive styles, and problem resolution to do with the question of why females may be put at-risk for anorexia? The connection derives from two observations based upon logic and evidence. Logic dictates that psychological defenses may be detrimental to the extent the temporary escape from the unpleasant emotions of stress makes it less likely that the person will attempt direct action against the source of stress as a way of resolving a personal problem. The second observation, based upon evidence from our research into defensive styles, is that the more effectively a preferred defense shuts people off from acknowledging a stressor, the more stress they report in their daily lives. These two observations, considered together, make a lot of sense. The further we defensively sidestep a source of stress, the less likely we are to deal with the stress at its source; failure to act directly upon a source of stress allows it to continue its contribution to our day-to-day stress burden.

Consider the four defensive styles in terms of how effectively they could circumvent a stressor, what I shall call "evasiveness." Rationalization involves directly dealing with the origin of stress and altering meaning in what may be only a modest way to make the information more tolerable. This in my mind is the least evasive strategy; the rationalizer maintains awareness of the more tolerable stressor for potential action. Studies have agreed that an emphasis upon rationalization as a defense is accompanied by low levels of daily stress (Heilbrun & Pepe, 1985; Heilbrun & Renert, 1988). At the most evasive extreme, repression represents putting the stressor "out of mind" by forgetting it; a stressor cannot be resolved by direct action to the extent it remains beyond awareness. This repressive tactic for relief from stress has been associated with the highest stress levels in our studies (Heilbrun & Pepe, 1985; Heilbrun & Renert, 1986). Projection and denial as defenses assume intermediate status as far as evasiveness is concerned and have been associated with intermediate levels of stress in these studies. Neither of these strategies of defense puts the stressor out of reach. Both defenses involve review of the stressful information before attempting to neutralize its unacceptable qualities through what could amount to rather gross distortions of reality.

Let me summarize this discussion of psychological defenses and solution of stress-promoting problems. The degrees of evasiveness implicit in the four major strategies lend themselves to a predicted order of procrastination in dealing with personal problems. The amount of stress reported by college students committed to these defenses confirm the same order suggesting that procrastination in dealing with problems allows them to continue taking an emotional toll. Repression makes it easiest to neglect the problem and ranks as the worst in these regards. Rationalization involves the least deterrent to problem-solving. Projection and denial fall in-between these extremes.

Evasiveness in contending with sources of stress can be influenced in many ways besides choice of defensive style. Two represent further twists of cognition that may complement the defenses and have received attention within our research. These additional cognitive traits included, for one, the person's degree of awareness that she uses a given defense to ward off disquieting information. For example, repression as a defense is associated with high stress, but when the person also shows limited awareness of her repressive style, stress level becomes even more extreme (Heilbrun & Pepe, 1985). Selectively forgetting a source of stress by forcing it from consciousness is evasive enough, but the less you are aware of what you have done, the further the source is put out of reach.

A superficial approach to information represents another facet of evasiveness that we have studied (Heilbrun, 1984; Heilbrun & Renert, 1986). The superficial individual settles for obvious and popular surface meanings. By dealing with information in a shallow rather than probing way, the person escapes alternative or associated meanings that could prove disquieting. Prejudice is more likely to thrive in those given to superficial thinking, since they are unlikely to question their simplistic conclusions. By the same token, superficial interpretations of experience could limit any real understanding of complicated problems that add stress to our lives. As understanding suffers, so would adequacy and permanence of solutions.

The use of repression as a defensive strategy, lack of awareness regarding the use of this strategy of defense, and a generally superficial approach to information, taken as a pattern, represent the most clearcut evidence of cognitive evasiveness by my analysis. The pattern would be detrimental to solving stress-provoking problems, since the problems would be shielded from resolution; a failure in resolution would expose the college woman to continuing stress and put her at greater anorectic risk.

A study by Heilbrun and Harris (1986) considered defensive style, level of awareness for the defenses, and superficiality among 53 college women sharing or relative free of anorectic characteristics. The high and low AP groups were formed by a median split of the sum scores for the six relevant EDI scales. Defense styles were measured by performance on a series of four standardized laboratory tasks on each of which instructions to the subject required her to engage in self-evaluation. Different defensive strategies were represented by each of the four tasks. The nature of task instructions, the task itself, and the rules of scoring the subject's self-appraisal made it possible to isolate and measure a particular style of defense on each component of the battery. That these measures are concerned with defensive styles is in no way obvious to the subject, allowing typical modes of defense to be displayed without demands made by research. The defensive-style tasks are fully described in nine research articles published between 1972 and 1986, cited on an earlier page. For present purposes, it may suffice to add that these tasks allow the person to utilize whatever styles of defense that come naturally. Defensive-style scores tend to be uncorrelated within a sample of subjects. Any given individual may show none, some, or all of the defenses in strength.

Awareness of defense was determined by comparing what the woman actually used in way of defense within the laboratory with ratings obtained from her at a later point in the study regarding her use of the same four defenses within her daily life. The ratings were based upon straightforward descriptions of the defenses, and the woman was advised that they were neither necessary behaviors nor mutually exclusive. If she denied a particular defense but it showed up as a defense of choice in the laboratory, lack of self-awareness was indicated. Finally, superficiality was quantified by free association to a series of words. Available norms for college students (Palermo & Jenkins, 1964) allowed us to establish whether the woman's associated words tended toward the commonplace and popular or toward broader associations more unique to the individual. Commonplace and popular associations were taken as evidence of superficiality. More unique associations rather than commonplace meanings were considered an indication of interest in what is beyond the obvious.

Table 3.3 contains the defensive-style scores provided by high and low AP females. Two comparisons revealed significant differences. The repression comparison points to the greater use of this strategy by high AP females ($p < .05$); anorectic risk is associated with an especially evasive tactic of defense. The opposite finding was evident in the projection results, with high AP subjects less inclined to use this defense than were the low AP controls ($p < .05$). The projection results, which forecast a deficit in that style of defense for the high AP female, were not greeted with much interest in the 1986 publication. The compelling logic of these results occurred to me some time later as the research program generated addi-tional evidence about the female at anorectic risk. The self-preoccupation of the woman at-risk for anorexia, confirmed later in this chapter, would detract from her sensitivity to the social environment. The social-comparison process, that I have placed at the heart of projection, requires a special sensitivity to the social environment so that models for comparison would be available. The self-preoccupied woman is not a candidate for a projective style of defense. Repression, a totally insular defense, would be readily accessible to this woman no matter how self-preoccupied she might be.

The defense-awareness results were consistent with the view that females at-risk for anorexia are not only especially evasive with regard to their defense against distressing information, but they are also self-deceptive with regard to use of the repressive defense. Both the distribution of laboratory-based repression scores and the distribution of ratings concerning actual use of repression were cut at their sample medians. Some 50% of the high AP females who were repressors in the laboratory (above the sample median) were unaware that they use repression (below the median rated use). Controls high in the use of repression provided a far lower unawareness figure of 22% ($p < .05$). No discrepancy in awareness between the two AP groups was found for the remaining three defenses.

At-risk subjects and their low AP controls, broken down further by the sample median on the repression score, were then compared in terms of their adherence to the commonplace in free association. High AP women, prone to using a repressive strategy of defense, were more

Table 3.3   Defenses in College Females with and without Anorectic Characteristics

	Females with Anorectic Characteristics (N = 28)	Females without Anorectic Characteristics (N = 25)
Defensive Style	M	M
Repression	51.29	44.64
Projection	44.96	51.80
Rationalization	51.29	51.08
Denial	49.50	49.68

Note. - Adapted from Heilbrun, A. B., & Harris, A. (1986). Psychological defenses in females at-risk for anorexia nervosa: An explanation for excessive stress in anorexic patients. International Journal of Eating Disorders, 5, 503-516.

superficial than AP subjects not given to repressive defenses. The opposite pattern was found for controls. The low AP woman's use of repression was combined with a more reflective approach to meaning that presumably would compensate for repressive tendencies. The opposite-direction findings were verified statistically by a significant interaction effect ($p < .05$).

Overall, then, the college women in the Heilbrun and Harris study who displayed some degree of risk for anorexia in their symptom picture included a subset at special risk because of a coalescence of cognitive qualities that would keep disturbing information at a distance. This was demonstrated in their use of repression, a highly evasive defense; unawareness of this preferred defense thereby making retrieval even more difficult; and a generally more superficial response to the meaning of information. There was no comparable coalition of evasive qualities in low AP females. Such broad cognitive evasiveness for the at-risk woman would offer some protection from stress on a temporary basis. At the same time, it would contribute to procrastination and poor problem resolution when she is faced with developmental problems relating to achievement, interpersonal distrust, and reluctance to assume adult roles. Problems kept out of mind are problems that are likely to continue as sources of stress.

Why Is Bodily Thinness Selected as the Compensatory Goal Substituting for Success in the Career or Interpersonal Domains?

Thinness as a value. We have considered the question of why problems involving competition for career and social achievement goals arise and persist as sources of stress for the high AP female. The next question becomes why a thin body assumes such priority as a substitute marker of achievement. The question may appear rhetorical to the reader, since a thin body has become such a common ideal among American women as to become the norm (Rodin et al., 1985). Given such consensus, departing from traditional opportunities for attainment and choosing thinness as a substitute goal might be expected to qualify as commonplace.

Even though the idealization of a thin body is the rule rather than the exception in women, there are still degrees of importance as with all values. That is probably why the Drive for Thinness scale was developed for the EDI, allowing for individual differences rather than assuming a universal preference for thinness. That the test developers were correct in assuming differences between women can be demonstrated very simply by post hoc analysis of data from the Heil-brun and Putter (1986) study of gender schemas. After dividing the sample of 69 college women into three levels based upon their Drive for Thinness scores alone, the discrepancy between ideal weight and actual weight was determined for the groupings. The third with the highest Drive for Thinness scores selected ideal weights averaging 15.07 pounds less that their actual weights. The middle third chose ideal weights 8.75 pounds under their current weights, and the third with the lowest scale scores had an average ideal only 3.38 pounds less than actual weight. The Drive for Thinness scale does identity some college women who hold out a much thinner body as an ideal, but the majority are more conservative in their body preference. The dis-crepancy between actual and preferred weight for the upper third of the scorers on Drive for Thinness cannot be explained in terms of current overweight, by the way. Generally speaking, these were not grossly overweight women wishing to approximate the norm. There are simply some college women who idealize thinness to an extreme and many others who are variably less committed to this value.

Femininity, preference for thinness, and anorectic risk. Evidence considered previously revealed that traditional feminine behavior, along with sensitivity to traditional sex-role expectations, tended to be associ-ated with higher anorectic risk in college women. The expressive character of traditional femininity, as it restricts female competi-tiveness, helps explain problems within usual achievement domains. I could just as readily use this evidence on femininity in college women to explain the high value placed upon a svelte body and the commit-ment to thinness as a substitute goal in those at anorectic risk. A thin female body has been identified as a feminine trait (Guy, Rankin, & Norvell, 1980) and dieting has been proposed as a feminine option (Hawkins, Turrell, & Jackson, 1983; Squires & Kagan, 1985). The longstanding cultural association between femininity and beauty in women (Rodin et al., 1985) and the critical role of thinness within the concept of female beauty in Western societies again draws a connection between femininity and thinness.

Traditional femininity may play a dual role as an anorectic risk fac-tor, then. Femininity and cognizance of traditional role behaviors could contribute to the development of achievement problems by interfering with competitive motivation. Being feminine and sensitive to tradition also could help explain the special value placed upon thinness that encourages goal substitution.

Self-preoccupation, preference for thinness, and anorectic risk.
Self-preoccupation will assume more than its share of importance as a
risk factor for anorexia nervosa as well as for the other stress-related
disorders to be considered later in the book. Self-preoccupation not
only contributes directly to the risks posed by dieting behaviors but
also seems to have referred risk effects. By this I mean that it seems to
foster other cognitive traits that in their turn contribute to food restraint
and to anorectic risk.

At this point, I am interested in considering one aspect of self-
preoccupation -- the at-risk woman's concern with food effects upon her
body and whether this is linked to an idealization of thinness. Both the
woman's preoccupation with food effects and the priority she assigns to
thinness appear to be important as far as explaining success on a diet,
perhaps too much success. The evidence to be reported here derives
from the work of Heilbrun and Flodin (1989), although the particular
analyses were not included in the published paper. The full set of
results covered by the Heilbrun and Flodin paper will be provided in
the next chapter when stress is introduced as a standard feature of our
studies into anorectic risk.

Heilbrun and Flodin developed a set of self-rating scales that
inquired into the eating attitudes and behaviors of female college subjects. Two of these ratings related directly to preoccupation with the
effect of food upon the body. One 5-point scale concerned how much
the subject thought about a gain in body weight as she prepared to eat
food. The second 5-point rating considered body perception after
eating by asking the extent to which the woman thought about appearing heavier after having eaten a meal. A third 5-point scale inquired
into body preoccupation and eating more indirectly by a query regarding degree of self-consciousness when the subject ate in public. We
hoped to pick up on how presumed and unwanted body changes or
simply the act of eating itself might be special concerns if viewed by
others. The sample of 68 females was split by the median EDI score
into high AP and control (low AP) groups. The three sets of ratings
were also divided into those above the sample median and those below
in preparation for nonparametric analysis (frequency counts).

The self-preoccupation ratings revealed that 61% of the high AP
women reported a greater preoccupation with increased body size
before eating. These at-risk females showed greater concern with
weight gain after eating was completed in 61% of the cases as well.
Only 17% of the control women admitted high self-preoccupation with

their bodies before or after eating. High self-consciousness when eating in public was reported by 45% of the high AP females and 17% of the controls. All frequency differences between AP and control groups were significant ($p < .05$). These figures show females symptomatically at-risk for anorexia nervosa to far more likely be preoccupied with the effects of food on their bodies before they eat or after they eat. Self-consciousness also appears to be a much more prevalent response among high AP women to eating in a public place where their bodies and their consumption of food would be on display.

Female concerns about increasing body size that appear before or after eating bear a logical relationship to their idealization of thinness. Analysis of the relationship between the ratings of body preoccupation before and after eating (added together) and the discrepancy between actual and ideal weight reported by the Heilbrun and Flodin college women supports this logic but not without complication. High AP women with greater (above the sample median) bodily self-preoccupation associated with eating demonstrated a remarkable deviation from their ideal weight. Their actual weight exceeded their personal ideal by 17.04 pounds. The few high AP women who lacked bodily preoccupation (below the median) revealed little discrepancy between actual and ideal weight (a .78 pound difference). These effects found in at-risk women follow the dictates of logic. The more a woman prizes a body far thinner than her own, the greater should be her preoccupation with food and its effect upon her body.

However, low AP controls did not display this logical relationship between a desire for a thin body and preoccupation with how food affects the body. Those whose self-ratings reflected greater concern with changes in body weight associated with eating and those who denied much concern were about the same in their idealization of thinness -- 10.24 pounds versus 7.72 pounds difference in actual and ideal weight, respectively. Statistical analysis verified the inconsistent nature of the relationship between food-inspired body preoccupation and discrepancy between actual and ideal weight. Higher and lower levels of preoccupation were associated with divergent average departures from ideal weight of 17.04 and .78 pounds, respectively ($p < .01$), within the high AP group. The counterpart discrepancies of 10.24 and 7.72 pounds for low AP women lacked significance when compared. That these controls showed no relation between body preoccupation associated with eating and how much they idealized thinness runs counter to my sense of logic, but in its own way helps clarify the anorectic risk picture. Women at low risk share the general disposition of college females to want a thinner body. However, they are far less likely to pair preference with the urgency implied by preoccupation with food, eating, and added girth.

The conclusion to be drawn from these analyses seems inescapable. Women at-risk for anorexia nervosa not only tend to be preoccupied with the danger of adding fat to their bodies by eating, but this body preoccupation is bolstered by a yearning for a much thinner body than they have. Both may serve as psychological restraints upon eating and both coalesce within the high AP female. Since these concerns relating to body size converge only in the high AP group and not in controls, we have another answer to the question of why bodily thinness is selected as a compensatory goal in women inviting the risk of anorexia nervosa. The psychological pattern including both idealization of thinness and body preoccupation makes it more likely that dieting will be attempted and, if attempted, will be successful. One without the other would provide a less formidable set of dieting credentials. This theme will reappear in the chapter to follow when I report research that bears upon the trademark feature of anorectic risk -- the coalescence of psychological factors that overdetermine the woman's ability to restrict her eating. In a real sense, she puts herself in danger of being victimized by her own success at dieting.

Chapter 4

Stress and the Risk of Anorectic Disorder: Studies of Individual Risk Factors

The research described in the previous chapter offers some insight into the personality factors that may introduce the risk of anorectic development. These not only help explain the lack of success in standard achievement domains but why the female so avidly seeks bodily thinness through dieting as a substitute for limited achievement. Not only do these setting factors cast light on body thinness as a chosen goal but begin to explain why a woman may place herself at greater risk of anorexia nervosa by not only reaching her goal but going beyond healthy limits.

The present chapter will turn to additional research that will focus more specifically upon the extraordinary success of food restraint that elevates anorectic risk and upon the role of stress in the risk pattern. Many college women may seek body thinness through dieting and place value upon achieving this goal, but only a few can be expected to go to such extremes as the anorectic. The difference is in the woman's vulnerability to distortions of perception and attention that serve her need for attaining a thin body. These distortions, along with heavy stress, will be considered as specific risk factors.

Perceptual Distortion, Stress, and Anorectic Risk

The research that will be summarized in this chapter was guided by a simple strategy. First, identify deviant cognitive qualities that would assist the woman in reaching her goal of a thin body through successful dieting but make it difficult to keep the process within reasonable limits. Then determine whether these cognitive distortions are related to the risk of anorexia nervosa as indicated by an anorectic profile. Finally, introduce stress into the evidence in such a way as to confirm its critical role as a complementary and necessary anorectic risk factor.

Three types of deviant cognition qualified in a clearcut way as vital to a level of food restraint that not only allows the woman to avoid eating in the face of hunger and temptation but to maintain this restraint until she reaches a dangerous level of emaciation. The most obvious deviant cognitive quality was body-image distortion, the perception of one's own body as fatter than is realistically the case. This type of anomalous perception would be important as a ready source of motivation for initiating or continuing a diet in someone with an aversion to a fat body. It is also a paramount symptom of anorexia nervosa which alerted me to its possible importance at the developmental stage of the disorder. Another perceptual quirk that might prove invaluable in bypassing food is the sense of an expanded body size brought on by the mere presence of food cues. Simply thinking about food or being in the presence of food would promote a sense of having a bulkier body. What better way to refrain from eating than to feel fatter just contemplating food? The third type of advantage in dieting would be gained by a failure in attention -- not experiencing hunger sensations to the extent most people do. If you do not feel hungry, then it is a lot easier to not eat.

Body-image distortion, stress, and anorectic risk. As I have said, a distorted body image is used as a defining symptom of anorexia nervosa according to the Diagnostic Manual. However, the research evidence regarding this perceptual anomaly is not as compelling as we would be led to expect. Earlier studies reported by Slade and Russell (1973) found that anorectics markedly overestimated their body widths relative to controls. Later review of the evidence by Slade (1985) led him to conclude that body overestimation could be found in a variety of female groups; anorectics were most prone to overestimate, however. In a more recent review of the literature, Whitehouse, Freeman, and Annadale (1988) found no difference between anorectics and controls in the way they perceived their bodies. Their own study substantiated this conclusion, although they did note that the anorectic subjects included some given to marked overestimation and others who grossly underestimated body size.

These three literature reviews offer contrasting versions of the importance of body-image distortion and an unrealistic sense of fatness as a symptom in anorexia nervosa. One tells us that the distorted perception of the anorectic is unique among women, the next that it is an exaggeration of a general trend, and the third that anorectics overall are not distinguishable from normal women in this regard. I believe that the rather erratic nature of these findings bearing upon the importance of body perception in anorexia could be explained if the functional role that body-image distortion plays in dietary restraint were considered along with the timing factor within the developmental history of the disorder. Once the anorectic reaches the attention of helping professionals in the hospital and is labeled a "patient," she has attained skeletal thinness and some degree of aversion to food. Perceiving herself as unrealistically fat at this stage of full-blown disorder may be less crucial to sustaining eating restraint than it was earlier when symptoms were developing. When researchers sample anorectics from patient populations for body-image studies, they may well have to contend with a less reliable perceptual effect. The symptom is there for some but not for others, because the body image no longer plays a crucial role in achieving or maintaining thinness.

Perceived enhancement of body size should represent a more important dynamic during an earlier period in anorectic development before dieting has gained a major foothold in the woman's life and when continued food restraint remains a matter of more tentative resolve. In other words, the motivational contribution of body-image distortion should be at its greatest when it is most needed to promote and sustain dieting behavior. Furthermore, our research will consider whether the critical role of body-image distortion may depend upon actual body size as well as developmental timing. It could be reasoned that the female with a thinner body who is driven to compensatory dieting by perceived achievement failure may experience a special problem in dealing with reality; her body is less in need of food restraint in order to meet the standards of thinness she embraces. This slimmer woman may need a motivational boost from a fattened body image to institute dieting or remain on a diet during the risk stage of the disorder. On the other hand, heavier women may have experienced special difficulties in food-restraint or view themselves realistically as having further to go in achieving their ideal weight. The motivational increment from a distorted body image could prove helpful in either case.

Our first inquiry into body imaging in college women (Heilbrun & Friedberg, 1990) applied the at-risk research method to 100 college females. AP status was determined from the EDI using a median-split procedure. The subject's body image was obtained in the following way. Alone with the female experimenter, she was asked to examine herself in a full-length mirror using both front and profile views. She then rated her body size along a 10-inch line labeled "very thin" at one end and "very fat" at the other. Body image was defined by the distance along the line measured to the nearest hundredth of an inch. This procedure was repeated after 10 minutes of filler activity to increase reliability of the measure. The final body-image score was represented by the average of these two highly correlated ratings.

Distorted body image was measured in this study by the Body Perception Index (BPI), proposed by Slade and Russell (1973). The BPI offered a straightforward mathematical formula for determining who was and who was not subject to distortion:

$$BPI = \frac{\text{average perceived size of body}}{\text{actual size of body}} \times 100$$

In order to use this formula, two arithmetic conversions were introduced. First, we wanted to increase the precision of this index, so a means of calibrating actual body proportions was adopted that improved upon using weight alone. The woman's weight in pounds was divided by her height in inches to represent how weight was distributed over the body frame. A woman weighing 140 pounds at 70 inches in height presents a very different body-size appearance than another woman at the same weight but reaching only 60 inches in height. Then both the body-image and actual body-size scores were converted to standard score distributions with a mean of 50 and standard deviation of 10 before they were introduced into the BPI formula. BPI scores exceeding 100 reflect body images that exaggerate actual body size relative to other women in the sample; scores less than 100 indicate degrees of underestimation, again relative to others in the sample. Although perceptual error can be in either direction, I shall reserve the term "distortion" for errors of overestimation on forthcoming pages.

Table 4.1 presents BPI scores for the sample of females after they had been subdivided by median AP score and into actually fatter and thinner groups by the median weight/height score. Statistical tests tell us that high AP women inflated their body images more than AP con-

Table 4.1   Body-image Scores for Women Sharing (High AP) and Not Sharing (Low AP) Anorectic Characteristics and Having Fatter and Thinner Actual Body Sizes

	High AP Women		Low AP Women	
Actual Body Size	N	M	N	M
Fatter	28	93.64	21	92.24
Thinner	22	118.55	29	103.83

Note. - The mean body weights in pounds for these four groups were: Fatter high AP = 133.78, fatter low AP = 134.62, thinner high AP = 112.05, and thinner low AP = 113.62. Adapted from Heilbrun, A. B., & Friedberg, L. (1990). Distorted body image in normal college women: Possible implications for the development of anorexia nervosa. Journal of Clinical Psychology, 46, 398-401.

trols ($\underline{p}$ < .005), and thinner women distorted their body images more than fatter women ($\underline{p}$ < .001). However, the one thing that stands out on this table is the singular degree of body-image distortion displayed by one group of women -- those who were thinner and had a higher anorectic profile. Their BPI scores were markedly elevated ($\underline{M}$ = 118.55), well in excess of the 100 index standard and indicating gross overestimation of body size. This elevated BPI score was reliably higher than any of the remaining three group means ($\underline{ps}$ < .001).

It is clear, then, that perceptual distortion as an early risk factor was found only in thinner college women who are beginning to display the behaviors associated with anorexia nervosa. These thinner women would seem to require the motivational boost of an inflated body image in order to initiate or sustain a diet. High AP women with heavier proportions did not evidence perceptual distortion as a risk factor; if anything, they tended to underestimate their girth.

The understanding of anorectic risk as evolving from a crisis of failing competition for achievement would lead us to expect that only college women who are under excessive stress would be at greater risk. Elevated stress would authenticate a troubled adjustment to the competitive environment and help explain the woman's motivation and strength of resolve in achieving a substitute goal as a way of bringing stress into line. Heilbrun and Friedberg chose to test the importance of stress as a source of vulnerability to anorexia nervosa by examining its level in women already at special risk because they combine the two other psychological risk factors under study -- high AP status and the presence of a distorted body image. Two questions will be raised within this analysis, each requiring the same result if it is to be answered in the theoretically affirmative way. One bears upon whether the troubled adjustment of the at-risk college woman can be verified by a singularly high level of stress. The other concerns whether the three risk factors -- high AP status, body-image distortion, and high stress -- coalesce into a single pattern of anorectic vulnerability.

This would be an opportune spot to introduce the reader to the stress measure that will be a standard feature of the research to be reported throughout the remainder of the book. Our interest was in using a response-based measure that would inquire into the amount of stress being experienced in the daily lives of our subjects. Other stress measures were available, but they lacked the focus we were seeking. Stimulus-based approaches emphasized the presence of situations in the subject's life in which stress would be expected, but these measures have some critical limitations in assessing actual stress loads. Some normally stressful situations may have little impact on a given woman, or the woman may be facing some unique sources of stress that are not represented among those selected by the test developer. There are, of course, ways in which these limitations can be countered psychometrically, but a response-based measure circumvents them entirely. Physiological stress measures (e.g., blood pressure) seemed too bound to the situation and time of measurement and less promising as an index of life stress. In keeping with these considerations, a new stress measure was devised for our research programs (Heilbrun & Pepe, 1985).

The measurement of stress symptoms was based upon the compilation of indicators proposed by Selye (1976), a pioneer among stress researchers. These indicators included numerous biological and behavioral signs of stress that would be readily apparent to the individual and available for self-report. Twenty-five symptoms were selected as most commonplace and appropriate for young-adult college students including such indicators as a racing heartbeat, dry mouth, emotional tenseness, nervous mannerisms, concentration problems, sleeping problems, frequent need to urinate, or headaches.

The symptoms are presented to the subject who is asked to rate how frequently each has been experienced over the span of the previous year. Ratings may extend from denial of the symptom at one extreme (score = 0) to experiencing the symptom on a more-than-daily basis (score = 5) at the other extreme. The 0 to 5 scoring for each symptom allows for a range of stress scores from 0 at the low end to 125 at the high extreme when summed. College subjects who have volunteered for my research over the years have provided scores that covered almost all of that range.

With a description of the stress-symptom measure behind us, we can proceed to the stress data provided by Heilbrun and Friedberg. Table 4.2 includes stress levels reported by high and low AP college women who overestimated their body size (BPI >100) or underestimated it (BPI < 101).

Statistics verified the presence of two overall effects in the stress data that serve as a prelude to the critical results. High AP women reported more stress than their controls ($p < .01$); women who inflated their body images received higher stress scores than women who underestimated their body size ($p < .01$). In other words, each risk factor was associated with elevated daily stress. Attention is drawn,

Table 4.2.   Stress Reported by High and Low AP Females Who Enhance or Diminish Their Body images

	High AP Females		Control Females	
Body Image Relative to Actual Body Size	$\underline{N}$	$\underline{M}$	$\underline{N}$	$\underline{M}$
Enhanced	30	58.27	19	45.05
Diminished	20	47.20	31	40.48

Note. - Unreported data taken from Heilbrun, A. B., & Friedberg, L. (1990). Distorted body image in normal college women: Possible implications for the development of anorexia nervosa. Journal of Clinical Psychology, 46, 398-401.

however, to the one group who received stress scores well in excess of any other group (all $ps < .05$). Women at-risk because of their anorectic profiles and because they distort their body images described their lives as most stressful. Within my understanding of anorectic risk in which stress serves as a bellwether of unresolved problems and as motivation for a substitute achievement goal, this finding both substantiates the developmental dilemma posed by preanorectic problems, achievement among them, and qualifies stress as an additional coalescing risk factor.

As is inevitably true for psychological research that seeks to explore complicated behavioral issues, many questions remain unanswered or are actually raised by the Heilbrun and Friedberg findings. Accordingly, the initial probe of body-image distortion, body size, and stress as risk factors was followed by a second study (Heilbrun & Witt, 1990) which attempted to resolve at least some of these questions about the role played by perception in fostering anorectic risk. First and foremost, we wanted to know whether the Heilbrun and Friedberg results could be replicated with a new sample of women. In addition, we were interested in exploring as best we could whether body-image distortion should be considered a part of the actual dynamics of anorectic development at a preclinical stage or simply as a sign of danger ahead without dynamic properties.

Two issues left unsettled by the first body-image study relating to the role of distortion in the dynamics of anorectic risk were chosen for follow-up investigation. Is the overestimation of body size found in thinner women with anorectic profiles an isolated perceptual distortion? The alternative would have body-size enhancement as part of a broader perceptual style which leads the woman to generally overestimate the size of objects in her environment. This is important in that an isolated body-image distortion out of character with the woman's usual way of viewing her environment would argue for the special impact of her need for food restraint upon perception. The woman's isolated overestimation of her body size seemingly would exist for the specific purpose of spurring on her dieting. If the body-image distorter views everything as larger than is really the case, the dynamic linkage with an anorexia-related drive for thinness tends to go out the window.

The second unresolved issue left as a legacy from the Heilbrun and Friedberg study was whether the findings involving body-image distortion and actual body size and their motivational implications could be applied to practical everyday experience. As was just discussed, we presumed a motivational role for distorted body image when it was found in a woman already at-risk for anorectic development. This became an even stronger conviction when the evidence showed that extraordinary body-image distortion was displayed only by high AP subjects whose actual body size was on the thinner side of the sample mid-point. Commitment to dieting in women who are already relatively thin would seem to be more tenuous and in need of a psychological boost. Perceiving themselves as fatter than they are would satisfy that need. The untested assumption here is that these thinner high AP women actually use body images as part of their strategy of dieting -- that distortion plays an active role in enhancing food restraint.

The pattern of means revealed in Table 4.3 clearly replicates the earlier Heilbrun and Friedberg (1990) findings. We repeated the identical research procedures with 50 new college women and found thinner females with high anorectic profiles perceived their bodies as unrealistically heavier than any other group (all $ps < .05$). The BPI scores ($M = 115.50$) of women who were both high AP and thinner, relative to the sample medians, suggested gross body-image distortion, and contrasted with the general tendency to underestimate body size in the remaining groups ($Ms = 92.64$-99.38). Perceptual distortion, as before, was shown to be the unique domain of the at-risk female whose own actual thinness could present a motivational problem for initiating or continuing food restraint.

The question of whether body-image distortion is part of a general tendency to overestimate the size of things or is an isolated perceptual anomaly for the at-risk woman was considered by obtaining ratings of size for eight inanimate objects. Photographs of common objects in our environment -- automobiles, fruit, house furniture, and vases -- were rated as thin to fat on the same kind of 10-inch lines used by the subjects to judge the size of their own bodies. These eight individual ratings (two objects within each category) were summed for the subject to give an overall object-image score. It was not necessary to use the index procedure involved in comparing body images, since each object rated was realistically the same size for all subjects, and no correction was required. The same AP level x thinner/fatter groups reported in Table 4.3 were compared with respect to general object-image score without a hint of difference. Thinner women at-risk for anorexia did not perceptually enhance the size of inanimate objects as they had the size of their own bodies. Finding object distortion only when their body images were considered suggests that the perception of the thinner high AP woman has been selectively influenced by her need to restrain

Table 4.3   Body-image Distortion in College Women With and Without Anorectic Characteristics Further Subdivided by Fatter and Thinner Body Sizes

Body Size	Women with Anorectic Characteristics		Women Without Anorectic Characteristics	
	$\underline{N}$	$\underline{M}$	$\underline{N}$	$\underline{M}$
Fatter	11	95.64	14	92.64
Thinner	12	115.50	13	99.38

Note. - Adapted from Heilbrun, A. B., & Witt, N. (1990). Distorted body image as a risk factor in anorexia nervosa: Replication and clarification. <u>Psychological Reports, 66</u>, 407-416.

food intake. This makes it easier to argue that body-image distortion plays a motivational role in preanorectic dynamics.

Procedures for analyzing the motivational role played by body-image distortion in strategies of dieting, our stab at practical application, were dictated by the limited number of college subjects available for analysis. I failed to gather a large sample to begin with and subsequently lost nine of the 50 subjects for this analysis who denied ever using a diet. The remaining 41 subjects were asked to rate the extent to which they had used each of five different strategies for losing weight along 5-point rating scales extending from "never depend upon this" (=1) to "always depend upon this" (=5). They also were asked to consider how well each of these strategies had worked for them in their efforts to diet; four-point scales were provided extending from "poorly" (=1) at one end to "very well" (=4) at the other.

The following five dieting strategies and their descriptions were provided to the subject for her ratings:

- (a) <u>Self-monitoring</u> or keeping an eye on your body to motivate continued weight loss
- (b) <u>Comparison</u> or comparing your body to someone else who has an enviable body shape
- (c) <u>Will power</u> or firm adherence to planned food intake
- (d) <u>Hunger suppression</u> or using chemical aids that reduce hunger
- (e) <u>Nibbling</u> or eating a little food several times a day to prevent hunger.

The first two dieting strategies require the person to make reference to her own body; either method would allow a distorted body image to play a motivational role in continued dieting. Rating values for these two strategy ratings were added to provide a "body-oriented" strategy score. The remaining three methods do not in themselves involve the person's reference to her own body. These "body-free" strategies also were combined into a single score. The predictions in this analysis were clearcut. If a distorted perception is to play a motivational part in actual dieting, we would expect a woman with an inflated body image (1) to place special emphasis upon body-oriented strategies and (2) to report that these strategies are more effective for her.

The composition of Table 4.4 illustrates the compromise required by subject limitation mentioned previously. We did not follow the usual practice of breaking the subjects down into AP levels, nor did we use body size as an independent variable. Rather, the BPI indexing pro-

Table 4.4.   Use and Effectiveness of Body-oriented and Body-free Strategies of Dieting for College Women Differing in Perception of Their Own Bodies

		Strategies of Dieting			
		Body-oriented Strategies		Body-free Strategies	
		Use	Effectiveness	Use	Effectiveness
Body Image	N	M	M	M	M
Enhanced	14	8.79	5.93	8.29	5.43
Realistic	12	7.83	5.42	8.50	4.92
Diminished	15	6.07	4.13	7.07	5.00

Note. - Adapted from Heilbrun, A. B., & Witt, N. (1990). Distorted body image as a risk factor in anorexia nervosa: Replication and clarification. Psychological Reports, 66, 407-416.

cedure was employed to identify three body-imaging categories by a tripartite split of the distribution of scores: Enhanced (BPI > 106), realistic (BPI = 90-106), and diminished (BPI < 90). Dividing the 41 subjects in this way allowed us to evaluate the role played by a fattened distortion of body size in dieting relative to other ways of perceiving your body. Table 4.4 reports the average body-oriented and body-free strategy scores for dieting reported by these three body-image groups along with scores representing the effectiveness of these strategies.

The analysis of body-oriented strategy scores revealed significant effects across body-image groups. The use of body-oriented techniques during dieting was strongest in women who perceive themselves as unrealistically fat, weakest in women who diminish their body images, and realistic perceivers fell in-between ($p < .001$). The same result was noted when effectiveness scores were compared. Women who distort their body-images find body-oriented strategies of dieting to be most effective, realistic perceivers next, and those who view their bodies as unrealistically thin find strategies involving the body to be least conducive to effective dieting ($p < .05$).

These results actually confirm the importance of body imaging within the dieting process in two ways. That women who perceive themselves as unrealistically bulky use their bodies more as a reference and do this as an effective strategy of dieting are the effects I have emphasized. It is also important to note that perception of the body influences dieting strategy at the other extreme. Women who entertain body images that are unrealistically thin tend to ignore their bodies as a reference for dieting and report that body-oriented strategies do not work well for them.

Table 4.4 confirms the absence of systematic ordering when the use and effectiveness of body-free strategies were compared for the three body-image groups; statistical tests failed to confirm group differences. Although reference to her body as part of dieting is clearly related to the kind of body image the woman projects, the remaining strategies of dieting are not. Body image, as we measure it in the laboratory, certainly seemed to qualify as important to actual dieting behavior.

Even though these dieting-strategy results did not directly consider either anorectic profile or body thinness, it should not be forgotten that two independent studies have found what we called "enhancers" (BPI > 106) to be concentrated within the high AP, thin subset of women. A check on the 41 subjects in the analysis of dieting strategies confirmed this concentration. High AP women with thinner bodies received BPI scores above 106 in 67% of the cases, and only 17% provided "diminished" image scores below 90. These figures can be compared with the representation of enhanced body imaging within the remaining groups that ranged between 8% and 30% and diminished perceptions of the body that varied from 30% to 58%.

Food-cue induction of a distorted body image, stress, and anorectic risk. Perception, the meaning we assign to things or events, contributes to food restraint during the preclinical stage when the woman assumes a risk of anorexia nervosa. Overstating body size offers a source of motivation for dieting, especially important for women who are relatively thin and who were found to display this form of distortion to an extreme. The facts that this unrealistic distortion of body size was not found in the perception of other common objects and that it found its way into actual dieting strategies make it seem likely that body-image distortion is a dynamic part of the at-risk woman's need for an ultra-thin body.

Further thought on the matter suggested that a related perceptual idiosyncrasy might make its own contribution to food restraint and anorectic risk. Consider what happens when a weight-conscious person on a diet is exposed to the presence of food or even to the thought of food. In either case, food cues may tempt the person to eat if she is hungry and to violate her diet. Success in food restraint depends in part on whether she can prevent herself from eating when exposed to food, real or imagined.

One psychological mechanism that should help inhibit eating, given the presence of food cues, would be a tendency to perceptually distort the effect of food upon the body. If the weight-conscious person responds with an overblown perception about the fattening effects of food when exposed to such cues, that person will find eating to be even more objectionable than her cautious regimen would otherwise require. This form of perceptual distortion would provide an immediate motivational boost to food restraint and make it more possible to ignore the temptation to eat. While this form of distortion bears some similarity to the body-image phenomenon that was just considered, there is an important difference in principle. The present perceptual mechanism is triggered by food cues; body-image distortion is not dependent upon food cues and can be called upon anytime. Accordingly, the perception of increased body size in response to food cues would tend to occur on top of an already distorted perception of body size in the at-risk woman. Readers will not have to settle for a statement of independence in principle for these two perceptual mechanisms, however; evidence confirming their separate contribution to anorectic risk will be presented in the next chapter.

Heilbrun and Flodin (1989) investigated the food-cue-induced perceptual mechanism in a study of 100 college women. The effects of food cues upon body perception were evaluated by using two series of photographs selected from popular women's magazines that featured adult female models. The photographs contained no food cues and presented the models in full-bodied poses. These series of 10 photographs each had been selected from a larger pool of photographs after initial ratings of thin to fat body sizes had been obtained from female faculty and graduate students. Stable body-size estimates for each model were obtained by averaging across judges. The two series of photographs were constituted by selecting two matched models across a range of body sizes and assigning one to each series. This resulted, as you would expect, in two series of photographs almost identically matched for model size.

The usual at-risk methodology was utilized including the EDI and stress-symptom measures. Effect of food cues upon body perception was gauged by a laboratory procedure in which the woman was first asked to use a 5-point scale (from "very thin" to "very fat") to rate each of the 10 models in one of the series with regard to body size. No explanation was offered as to why these ratings were being collected. Once this series was completed and 10 minutes of filler activity had elapsed, the subject was requested to rate the body size of the models in the second matched series of photographs. Before she started the second series, four pictures of food taken from magazines were placed in plain view of the subject. The woman was told that they were to provide a context for judging the second series of models, since we were interested in the suitability of the models for food advertisements. The real purpose, of course, was to allow some loose association between food cues and the subject's perception of the female body in the second series of photographs.

Determination of how a subject was influenced by the presence of food cues in her perception of female body size was made by averaging the 10 ratings in the first series, made before food cues were present, and repeating this procedure for the second series of ratings obtained after food cues were introduced. If the average rating went up (in the fatter direction) for the second series, the subject was defined as an "enhancer," and the failure to view bodies as larger in the presence of food cues defined the "nonenhancer."

The strategy of analysis involved a median breakdown of the sample into high and low AP females, as usual, along with a sample subdivision into perceptual enhancers and nonenhancers. Stress level was subjected to analysis and became the yardstick of overall anorectic vulnerability shared by subjects in any particular group. This approach to analysis in which stress became the dependent variable was adopted for most of the studies in our program in which stress was measured. A singular elevation in stress was taken to mean that stress-generating problems were evident and the motivational basis for an anorectic solution had been identified. If peak stress scores were associated with other risk factors, in this case high AP status and body enhancement, the coalescence of risk factors would emerge as a pattern of heightened vulnerability to anorectic disorder.

The Heilbrun and Flodin paper also included the results of a replication study involving 68 additional college women. The methodology was identical to that described in the previous paragraphs except for a minor simplification of the presentation procedures for the photographs of female models. Table 4.5 presents the average stress reported by females, broken down by anorectic profile and body enhancement, for both the original and replication study.

The critical analysis in both studies revealed the same results. In the first study, perceptual enhancement of body size in the context of food cues for the high AP female was associated with peak stress relative to the high AP female who failed to show this form of perceptual distortion ($p < .05$). Stress scores obtained by enhancing and nonenhancing controls were low and much alike.

The replication study produced the same pattern of results, perhaps even more convincingly portrayed. Perceptual enhancers within the high AP group reported singularly high stress that exceeded high AP nonenhancers ($p < .001$), and enhancers and nonenhancers within the control group displayed the same low level of stress. Both studies, then, confirmed the coalescence of the three anorectic risk factors within a single subset of women. Those who indicated the emerging presence of anorectic symptoms by high AP scores and who perceived female bodies as fatter simply because food cues were introduced also were those reporting excessive stress.

The two studies I have just reported would have been even more compelling if the at-risk women's perception of their own bodies had been influenced by the introduction of food cues rather than the bodies

Table 4.5. Stress Reported by High and Low AP Females as a Function of Body-size Enhancement or Nonenhancement in the Presence of Food Cues (Initial and Replication Studies)

Perception of Body Size in Presence of Food Cues	Initial Study				Replication Study			
	High AP Females		Low AP Females		High AP Females		Low AP Females	
	N	M	N	M	N	M	N	M
Enhancement	20	56.85	28	37.43	19	54.37	14	36.57
Nonenhancement	26	46.54	26	36.81	21	35.24	14	36.57

Note. - Data taken from Heilbrun, A. B., & Flodin, A. (1989). Food cues and perceptual distortion of the female body: Implications for food avoidance in the early dynamics of anorexia nervosa. Journal of Clinical Psychology, 45, 843-851.

of photographed models. It is, after all, the perceived effect of food upon the person's own body that would be expected to most directly influence her eating. The choice of photographed models for this research was based upon methodological concerns regarding this perceptual variable that led me to seek the reliability of repeated subject observations of the female body. However, the importance of extending the body-enhancement findings to the at-risk female's perception of her own body led Heilbrun and Flodin (1989) to gather additional data in the replication study. Rating scales inquired into the effects of food stimulation upon the person herself as she entertained the thought of eating, experienced food actually eaten, or chose to eat in public. Evidence from these self-ratings has received attention on earlier pages when I considered self-preoccupation and idealization of thinness in terms of the woman's special concern for how food affects her body.

The following kinds of information were obtained from self-rating scales completed by the subjects in order to confirm perceived enhancement of the woman's own body, triggered by food cues, as a risk factor. Other items of interest relating to food, eating, and stress were subjected to rating as well. The items in the order presented to subjects were:

(a)   "When you prepare to eat food, do you have thoughts about how it will put weight on your body?" (5-point scale from "almost never" = 0 to "almost all the time" = 4)

(b)   "Do you ever think about how your body shape may have changed simply by having eaten a meal?" (5-point scale from "never think about looking a lot heavier = 0 to "often think about looking a lot heavier" = 4)

(c)   "How does being nervous and under stress affect your hunger for food?" (7-point scale from "makes me a lot less hungry" = -3 to "makes me a lot more hungry" = +3)

(d)   "Does eating affect how nervous and stressed you feel?" (7-point scale from "makes me feel a lot less nervous and stressed = -3 to "makes me feel a lot more nervous and stressed" = +3)

(e)   "Do you plan your food intake ahead of time?" (4-point scale from "never think about it ahead of time" = 0 to "sometimes the day before" = 3)

(f)   "If food is present at a social function does it make you

feel less social?" (4-point scale from "no difference" = 0
to "no difference" = 3)

(g)   "Are you self-conscious when you are eating in public?"
(4-point scale from "not self-conscious at all" = 0 to
"very self-conscious" = 3).

The effort to establish whether the replicated results from the
laboratory studies of perceived body distortion induced by food cues
would be found if the focus was shifted from photographed female
models to the female subject's own body proceeded along two lines.
First, ratings on scales a and b were summed for each subject to
estimate how much she perceived herself becoming heavier before and
after the ingestion of food. In either case, it can be safely assumed that
the woman is exposed to real or symbolic food cues. The correlation
between the sum score and the arithmetic change in body ratings for the
photographic models that defined enhancement or nonenhancement in
the two laboratory studies was then determined. This statistic will tell
us whether females who enhance other women's bodies once food cues
are introduced also tend to enhance their own body sizes when food
stimuli are in evidence. The correlation for the 33 high AP subjects in
the replication study was .34 ($\underline{p}$ < .05). There was a tendency for perceptual enhancement to occur in the presence of food cues for the at-
risk female whether other women's bodies or their own bodies were at
issue. The 35 control subjects failed to provide a significant correlation
($\underline{r}$ = -.24). In fact, if this nonsignificant negative correlation has any
meaning at all, it would suggest that these two types of body perception
tend to be at odds with each other in controls.

The female's perception of her own body in the context of food cues
also was subjected to analysis in a second way. The scales a and b sum
score was divided at its median; scores above the median defined own-
body enhancers. The high AP, own-body enhancers represented college
women at greatest risk in this particular self-report analysis. This key
group was examined in terms of the remaining food-related and eating-
related behaviors that appear relevant to anorectic risk. The ratings on
scales c through g will allow us to judge whether distorted perception
of food effects on her own body in the otherwise at-risk woman brings
with it other peculiarities associated with food and eating. The median-
split of the summed scores on rating scales a and b combined with the
existing high and low AP categories from the replication study provided the four subgroups on Table 4.6.

Statistical analyses of the five sets of ratings reported in Table 4.6

Table 4.6.   Food-related Experiences of High and Low AP Females Further Subdivided by Enhancement or Nonenhancement of their Own Body Size in the Presence of Food Cues

	High AP Females		Low AP Females	
	Enhancers ($\underline{N}$ = 17)	Nonenhancers ($\underline{N}$ = 16)	Enhancers ($\underline{N}$ = 17)	Nonenhancers ($\underline{N}$ = 18)
Rating Scale	$\underline{M}$	$\underline{M}$	$\underline{M}$	$\underline{M}$
Effect of eating on feeling stressed	.82	-.19	.12	.00
Planning food intake ahead of time	2.24	.81	1.12	1.11
Self-consciousness eating in public	1.76	1.19	.94	.61
Decreased sociability eating in public	.47	.25	.06	.17
Stress effect upon hunger	1.29	-.56	.88	.72

Note. - Adapted from Heilbrun, A. B. & Flodin, A. (1989). Food cues and perceptual distortion of the female body: Implications for food avoidance in the early dynamics of anorexia nervosa. Journal of Clinical Psychology, 45, 843-851.

revealed a remarkable consistency in that they warned of the eccentricities surrounding food and eating for college women otherwise at-risk for anorexia nervosa. These eccentricities of the at-risk woman not only emphasized a number of psychological mechanisms supporting food restraint but also offered some insight into why she must mobilize these mechanisms to get the job done. I will discuss these ratings in an order differing slightly from that presented to the subjects. The first set of findings found high AP, own-body enhancers reporting a uniquely elevated level of stress over eating (M = .82), above that of the high AP nonenhancers (M = -.19, p < .01). Own-body enhancement in the presence of food cues did not relate to eating-related stress within the control group; rating means were intermediate (.00-.12) and closely aligned for enhancers and nonenhancers. Therefore, the pattern of results involving AP status, perceptual body distortion, and stress was identical whether perception was directed to photographed models or the subject's own body and whether stress refers to total life experience or eating alone. In either case, a higher anorectic risk is indicated by the association of preclinical anorectic symptoms, a sense of a fattened body induced by food cues, and stress.

Self-reports bearing upon a number of other eating experiences revealed additional ways in which the high AP, own-body enhancer's concern about eating could deter food intake. The next three sets of ratings in Table 4.6 represent cases in point. The tendency to plan food intake ahead was more evident in the high AP enhancer (M = 2.24) than any other group, clearly exceeding the high AP nonenhancer (M = .81, p < .001). Whether the subject was or was not a body enhancer made no difference with regard to planned eating for control females (Ms = 1.11-1.12).

Eating in public resulted in the greatest self-consciousness for high AP enhancers (M = 1.76), more so than for her high AP counterpart who is not inclined to experience her body as larger in the presence of food cues (M = 1.19, p < .05). No effect of body enhancement upon self-consciousness was found among low AP women (Ms = .61-.94).

The question of whether eating in public actually decreased how sociable the woman felt failed to provide statistical differences among the groups when the statistical comparisons were made in the routine way. However, an alternative comparison in which high AP enhancers (M = .47) are compared to low AP enhancers (M = .06) did provide a small but significant finding that led to much the same conclusions. The high AP enhancer revealed decreased sociability when partaking of food in a public place relative to the low AP enhancer ($\underline{p}$ < .05). Nonenhancers, whether high AP or control ($\underline{M}$s = .17-.25), did not differ on this variable. Generally speaking, then, the woman who combines a high anorectic profile with a sense of her body becoming fatter when she eats or even thinks about eating also demonstrates the characteristics of the more obsessive dieter. She reports a more rigid planfulness concerning food and discomfort as shown by increased self-consciousness and decreased sociability when she eats around other people.

The final rating item (g) summarized within Table 4.6, if considered in combination with the first item (a), shows promise of explaining why some at-risk females must depend upon perceptual distortion that overstates the fattening effects of food as an added deterrent to eating. When asked what kind of effect stress had upon their hunger, high AP, own-body enhancers ($\underline{M}$ = 1.29) and nonenhancers ($\underline{M}$ = -.56) reported a rather striking difference ($\underline{p}$ < .001). Those who magnify their own body size in response to food cues indicated that stress increases their hunger, whereas nonenhancers reported that stress actually suppresses hunger. Controls who enhance ($\underline{M}$ = .88) and do not enhance body size ($\underline{M}$ = .72) provided similar ratings that fell in-between.

These stress-and-hunger findings allow for an intriguing possibility. They suggest a circular effect that could jeopardize a diet unless other psychological barriers to eating fell into place. High AP enhancers report far and away the greatest life stress (Table 4.5), and the first set of ratings in Table 4.6 makes reference to a special stress that derives from food cues, presumably based upon the temptation to eat or the actuality of having eaten. Given that much stress, the fact that this emotional state actually increases their hunger places the high AP, enhancing woman at special risk of breaching her dietary restraint. A circular effect seems almost inevitable; stress increases hunger and hunger-induced contemplation or consumption of food increases stress which, in turn, increases hunger. The at-risk woman exposed to this circular effect would have a special need for whatever assistance a distorted perception of her body could offer in an effort to counteract hunger and restrain eating. Anorexia nervosa literally means a loss of hunger having nervous origins (Slade, 1982). The present results suggest just the opposite is true during the at-risk stage of anorectic development when the vulnerable woman is beset by stress-enhanced hunger.

Disattention, Stress, and Anorectic Risk

As I stated in concluding the discussion of the ratings reported in Table 4.6, the perceptual distortion of body size found in women at-risk for anorexia nervosa qualifies as a deterrent to eating. Furthermore, the distortion may be necessary because of a psychobiological quirk; stress, in plentiful supply among women at anorectic risk, is associated with a sense of increased hunger in those who distort their body size. Distorted body images seem to be one way of combatting the increment in hunger and the instigation to eat. Any psychological trait that contributes to food restraint serves as a further source of vulnerability in females already at some anorectic risk. Whether we are considering ordinary body-image distortion or enhanced images of the body in the presence of food cues, it seems clear that the perceptual system is serving the weight-conscious woman's need to avoid eating and increasing her risk of disorder.

However, another possible source of vulnerability to anorexia nervosa resulting from the woman's response to stress and hunger can be identified outside of the perceptual system. The at-risk woman who is less aware of hunger sensations or is otherwise able to ignore them should be in a better position to restrain eating. No matter how strong the sensations of hunger, their failure to register in consciousness would make eating a less compelling choice and increase anorectic risk. Attention to the sensations of hunger became the next cognitive trait selected for at-risk investigation.

Inner turbulence and stress.   Heilbrun and Worobow (1990) reported two studies relevant to the issue of whether insensitivity to hunger sensations serves as a risk factor in anorexia. The first of these involved a microanalysis of the six anorectic scales featured by the EDI and making up the anorectic profile. Foremost among these scales for present purposes is Interoceptive Awareness. The 10 items in this scale involve two categories of experience that the test developers considered integral to anorexia nervosa. Some of them include content inquiring into the presence of strong inner sensations or the fear of being overwhelmed by such sensations. As examples, item #8 states, "I get frightened when my feelings are too strong."; item #44 offers, "I worry that my feelings will get out of control." Stronger endorsement of either statement approximates the anorectic experience.

The second type of item included on the Interoceptive Awareness scale considers the indistinctiveness of inner sensations that make it difficult for the anorectic to know exactly what she is feeling. Examples here would be: "I get confused about what emotion I am feeling." (item #20), and "I have feelings I can't quite identify." (item #60). It is obvious that the experts who developed the EDI viewed the anorectic as vulnerable to high levels of internal sensations and to problems in identifying their sources. This examination of EDI items encouraged us to believe that the poor quality of inwardly-directed attention might be involved as an anorectic risk factor.

Going beyond inspection of item content, however, we were interested in whether the inner turbulence and blunted sensitivity of the woman scoring high on the Interoceptive Awareness scale was related to the amount of stress reported in her daily life that places her at anorectic risk as I construe the development of the disorder. The question to be investigated became whether stress as one of our major risk factors fits into a more traditional diagnostic mold for anorexia nervosa. Can the inner turbulence be traced in important measure to an upsurge of stress?

Data analysis in the first Heilbrun and Worobow study considered the relationship between stress-symptom scores and Interoceptive Awareness for 100 college women. A correlation of .52 ($p < .01$) between stress and Interoceptive Awareness scores was obtained. This correlation suggests that stress does contribute substantially to the inner turbulence of the woman at-risk for anorectic development and to her resulting problems with identifying sources of inner stimulation. Hunger sensations must take their place within a sea of stimuli including the emotions of stress. The discrimination of hunger pangs as they are aroused would be expected to suffer for the at-risk woman as part of her general problem in identifying sources of stimulation within this turbulence.

Disattention to hunger sensations, reduced appetite, and anorectic risk. A second study, based upon a new sample of 80 college females, also was reported by Heilbrun and Worobow (1990). This investigation considered disattention to hunger sensations as a cognitive trait that would supplement the effects of faulty discrimination as a basis for disregarding hunger cues, reducing motivation to eat, and increasing anorectic risk. We believed it possible that the at-risk woman may display a specific cognitive deficit in attention to hunger sensations much like the insensitivity to hunger satiety cues that was found when women at bulimic risk were studied. The difference between these two risk-provoking deficits resides in their dynamic subtlety. A failure to be responsive to hunger sensations for the woman at anorectic risk readily qualifies as motivated behavior, since it serves an important goal of body thinness. In the case of insensitivity to satiety cues, the failure to stop binge eating satisfies no obvious purpose unless self-punishment is involved.

Disattention, as we used the term, represented a motivated effort to ignore a particular type of stimulation with the person more or less aware of this effort. This strategy of attention deployment is not particularly unusual. The attempt to exclude extraneous stimuli while studying or to ignore inner sensations of discomfort or pain would be commonplace examples of motivated disattention. A disattentional strategy can be contrasted with a simple failure of nearby stimulation to register in awareness. Motivated insensitivity requires something extra to make the strategy work such as concentrating on one stimulus in order to preclude awareness of another.

The sample of women was given the EDI along with Nideffer's measure of attentional styles. This attentional measure was introduced to the reader in the previous chapter as part of the study of satiety cues and bulimic risk when one of its scales was used to gauge effective focusing of attention. Our interest in the present study was directed towards another scale, Reduced Attentional Focus (RED). This 15-item scale portrays the narrowing of attention past some optimal point of effectiveness so that important information is lost. (Item #15 is, "I focus on one small part of what a person says and miss the total message.") RED approximates a general mechanism of disattention, although Nideffer does not introduce that term. A high score would suggest that the person focuses so hard on one point of stimulation that other cues are not noticed. This style of attention would allow the woman to further reduce the impact of hunger sensations and make food restraint an easier matter.

The first step in this multi-stage study considered the proposition that disattention in general was associated with anorectic risk. This served as a prelude to our more specific interest in disattention to hunger sensations as a risk factor. The sample of women was split into high and low AP groups by the usual median-split procedure. The RED scores for these two groups were then compared. A mean of 27.60 was found for the at-risk women as opposed to an average of 23.45 for the low AP females. Statistical test revealed a reliable ($p < .01$) difference between these scores. Encouraging further analysis of disattention, women at some anorectic risk did report a style of attention in which elements of a stimulus pattern tend to be excluded by overconcentration on some particular aspect.

Having found evidence that high AP females may be especially prone to selective attention, Heilbrun and Worobow turned to the next important set of questions. Does narrowing the focus of attention, as it would apply to inner stimulation, tend to restrict sensitivity to sensations of hunger for the at-risk AP woman. If this specific deficit in attention is found, are other kinds of sensations affected as well? If only hunger stimulation is influenced, motivated disattention could be assumed and another risk factor for anorectic development could be added with some confidence. Reduced attention to inner sensations of hunger, along with the generally faulty discrimination for all sources of stimulation from within, would limit the otherwise compelling effects of hunger.

The 80 college women in the second study were asked to complete a series of rating scales much like those described previously in the study of satiety cues in college women at-risk for bulimia (Heilbrun & Worobow, 1991). The scales included two types of ratings bearing upon subject sensitivity to hunger sensations. One scale was worded in terms of <u>awareness</u> of their occurrence. The second scale considered <u>responsive action</u>, the extent to which the hunger sensations were taken into consideration (by eating) when they did register or were simply ignored. Both scales presented the subjects rating points from a low of 1 to a high of 5. Awareness ratings offered choices from "unaware unless very strong" at the low end to "extremely aware" at the high end. Responsive action rating points extended from "try not to consider hunger sensations at all" to "take hunger sensations into consideration whenever they occur" at the extremes. Control ratings of awareness and responsive action were obtained for six other sources of inner sensation (pain, fatigue, thirst, boredom, emotions, and temperature) on the same type of scales.

The upper half of Table 4.7 includes the hunger-sensitivity rating scores for women with high anorectic profiles and low AP females, broken down further into high and low disattention groups by the median RED score. Statistical analysis of the hunger-awareness scores revealed an overall interaction ($p < .005$). This significant effect provided even more compelling results than we had reason to expect. On the one hand, we found a reduction in awareness of hunger sensations ($M = 3.21$) for women with high anorectic profiles who were also generally prone to disattention; women showing elevated AP scores but not inclined to disengage from stimuli by attentional means showed

Table 4.7.   Sensitivity to Hunger and Other Sources of Inner Sensations in College Females Having an Anorectic Profile and Controls as a Further Function of Disattention.[a]

Type of Inner Stimulation and Sensitivity to Sensations	Women With High Anorectic Profile		Control Women	
	High Disattention ($N = 28$)	Low Disattention ($N = 14$)	High Disattention ($N = 10$)	Low Disattention ($N = 28$)
	M	M	M	M
Hunger Sensations				
Awareness	3.21	4.00	3.90	3.36
Responsive Action	2.89	4.07	3.00	3.43
Residual Sensations				
Awareness	21.04	21.07	21.30	20.25
Responsive Action	20.00	19.71	18.80	20.21

Note. - Adapted from Heilbrun, A. B., & Worobow, A. L. (1990).   Attention and disordered eating behavior: II. Disattention to turbulent inner sensations as a risk factor in the development of anorexia nervosa. *Psychological Reports*, 66, 467-478.

[a]Based upon the Reduced Attentional Focus scale.

themselves to be more aware of hunger sensations ($\underline{M}$ = 4.00), $\underline{p}$ < .01. Disattention to hunger cues, which should decrease hunger and assist food restraint, emerged as a significant anorectic risk factor in a subset of women otherwise at-risk because of their high AP scores and general inclination toward selective attention. The rest of the interaction effect resulted from the failure to find this disattentional effect in the control women. In fact, the opposite was observed, although the reversal within the low AP group lacked statistical significance. Control women, not burdened by anorectic concerns, who reported general disattention were more aware of being hungry, if anything.

Considering next how the subjects described their responsiveness to hunger sensations, one critical effect was observed beyond the significant interaction ($\underline{p}$ < .005). Females already at anorectic risk because of their EDI profile and with a reduced focus of attention as an added risk factor reported being less responsive to hunger stimulation ($\underline{M}$ = 2.89) than high AP females not given to disattention ($\underline{M}$ = 4.07), ($\underline{p}$ < .001). No effect was found when low AP women were separated by level of attentional focus and compared on rated responsiveness. Again, disattention is identified as an anorectic risk factor at two levels of specificity but only in high AP women. This time high AP females who scored as generally disattentive on the RED scale reported a diminished response to feeling hungry, to whatever extent hunger sensations do register in awareness. Reduced response to hunger sensations that are detected, like reduced awareness of those sensations, would serve the goal of food restraint.

<u>Disattention as an isolated attentional risk factor in anorectic development</u>. The methodology of the Heilbrun and Worobow study of attention in anorectic development, as described to this point, has considered whether disattention as a risk factor is embodied in a generalized tendency to preclude aspects of a stimulus pattern from awareness or is restricted to a tendency to ignore hunger sensations. The answer seems to be that ignoring hunger cues is specific to high AP women, but this dynamic of food restraint is found only in those at-risk women who are generally inclined to disengage from any stimuli when they focus on an element of a pattern. General disattention breeds specific disattention to hunger sensations in females with an elevated anorectic profile.

In addition, the investigation considered whether disattention to internal sensations was a specific psychological mechanism aimed at hunger sensations for the at-risk woman or part of a more comprehensive attentional deficit affecting other sensations. This control analysis has a further bearing upon the confidence that can be invested in disattention as an anorectic risk factor. If it can be shown that the presence of a disattentional strategy in at-risk women only serves to attenuate sensitivity to hunger sensations and not other types of inner stimulation, it would provide a more compelling argument for the operation of a motivated attentional mechanism.

The ratings of awareness for the six sensations emanating from sources other than hunger were summed for each subject as were the responsive-action ratings. When these more general sensitivity scores were compared for the four AP x disattention groups (bottom half of Table 4.7), there was no hint of a difference among them. The reduced sensitivity to hunger sensations found for women at anorectic risk and generally inclined to disattend was not found when their sensitivity to six other types of inner sensations were considered. Disattention to inner stimulation appears to be restricted to hunger sensations for the at-risk woman.

A final comment about the data in Table 4.7 is in order before I move on to another analysis of isolated effects. It can be noted that general disattention as evidenced by elevated RED scores is more common in high AP women ($N = 28$) than its absence ($N = 14$), whereas high ($N = 10$) and low ($N = 28$) disattention have the opposite representation in low AP controls. These proportional differences, using the sample median as the reference point, are significant ($p < .001$). This disproportionality lends further confidence to the proposed defensive quality of reduced attention and to its conceptualization by the RED scale of the TAIS. I find it reassuring from a measurement perspective that high AP females display high disattention in two cases out of three; you would expect a strategy of attention that seems to make it possible to overlook hunger to be overrepresented in the at-risk group. Control women, not given to eluding hunger sensations, should include far fewer disattenders by RED standards; only 26% fell in the high disattention group.

Another type of evidence relevant to the issue of how isolated the disregard for hunger sensations might be in the disattentional woman at anorectic risk was made possible by the inclusion of two more ratings. These concerned the subject's sensitivity to hunger satiety cues and, as before, included the woman's <u>awareness</u> of these inner sensations and <u>responsive action</u> to them. We included these additional ratings, because our investigation of disattention might provide findings that seem at odds with those from another study of satiety sensations as a bulimic risk factor (Heilbrun & Worobow, 1991). You may recall that college women at higher bulimic risk reported less sensitivity to cues marking fullness than controls, and this allowed some explanation for binge eating. At the same time, when the same sample of women was reordered by anorectic risk, the difference in sensitivity to satiety cues disappeared as expected. However, this negative finding for women at anorectic risk presents a conundrum in light of the present results. Does it make sense to propose that women running the risk of anorexia nervosa would disattend to hunger sensations while at the same time they do not diminish their attention toward the complementary sensations of hunger satiation?

The average 5-point ratings on <u>awareness</u> of satiety cues for the four AP x RED disattention groups were as follows: Disattending and high AP women, $\underline{M} = 3.52$; attending and high AP women, $\underline{M} = 2.93$; disattending control women, $\underline{M} = 3.17$; and attending control women, $\underline{M} = 3.55$. Statistical comparison of the means provided a significant interaction ($\underline{p} < .05$) as the effect found in one sector of the data set appeared as an opposite effect in the other. You will notice that the women with high anorectic profiles who reported greater disattention showed an enhanced awareness of satiety signals, not a lesser awareness required by a disattentional strategy. Control women showed the opposite effect. The same arithmetic pattern of average ratings was obtained with <u>responsive action</u>, but the interaction fell short of significance.

While these satiety ratings are not robust, they are compelling as far as they go. The inconsistency between the reported insensitivity of the disattending, high AP female to sensations of hunger and sensitivity to satiety allows for but one conclusion. The effects of disattention are even more specific as far as internal sensations are concerned than I had thought. The high AP woman's withdrawal of attention only reduces her sensitivity to hunger sensations and not to other sources of stimulation. The sole affected sensation was the one that would threaten food restraint. The data now reveal that her sensitivity to sensations associated with eating that help her resist food remains intact. In fact, sensitivity to eating satiety cues qualified as relatively strong. This satiety evidence, combined with our findings on hunger sensations versus other sources of inner stimulation, argues strongly for a circumscribed effect of disattention to hunger sensations brought about by the high AP woman's need to avoid food and lose weight. It also argues strongly for the importance of motivated disattention as an anorectic risk factor.

This marks the end of my presentation of studies emphasizing individual cognitive factors that lend themselves to food restraint in stressed college females otherwise at-risk for anorexia nervosa. The evidence, in my opinion, presents a very credible case. Each perceptual or attentional factor considered independently implicated behavior that would contribute to food restraint and make the achievement of skeletal thinness a more likely reality. Consider the sheer number of these factors, and it becomes clear how the high AP woman can deter eating -- a distorted body image, preference for dieting strategies that involve reference to her perceptually-distorted body, sense of body fattening in the presence of food cues, cautious and unreceptive attitudes toward eating, emersion of hunger cues in a sea of other sensations including the emotions of stress, and specific disattention to hunger cues that might otherwise be detected. In the final chapter on anorectic risk, the emphasis will shift as we consider the extent to which the risk factors coalesce into patterns that imply even greater vulnerability.

Chapter 5

Stress and the Risk of Anorectic Disorder: Studies of Risk Patterns

The studies reported in Chapters 3 and 4 followed a fairly standard methodology in the search for evidence bearing upon the risk of anorexia nervosa. Each research effort involved two types of risk variables. One type included variables that are fundamental to the at-risk method for studying vulnerability to anorexia as a stress-related disorder. The endorsement of anorectic symptoms at some preclinical level and, later, the presence of extraordinary levels of stress appeared repeatedly across studies as basic markers of risk. The second type of variable involved new risk factors that would be tested individually by the verdict of empirical evidence, clinical judgment, and logic in each investigation. Examining one new cognitive/social risk factor per study seemed proper in the first stage of developing a network of anorectic risk variables when confirmation is paramount. However, it does not exploit the potential of the risk network that might follow from considering more than one of these new factors at a time.

My purpose in this chapter will be to consider both types of anorectic risk factors in extended combinations -- risk patterns of varying complexity. There are a number of questions regarding these patterns that might be of interest. One might wonder, simply as a matter of theoretical curiosity, whether the variables in a combination are related or even redundant when it comes to specifying risk. Some appear to be more closely aligned than others based upon similar behaviors that are involved (e.g., body-image distortion and body enhancement in the presence of food cues). This will not be a major focus, however, since my interest is more applied than theoretical at this point.

Greater priority will be given to the practical implications of coalescence for the risk factors. The question that matters for now is whether these variables converge into patterns that might improve our ability to identify the seriously at-risk individual? The convergence of risk factors represents a vital interest to anyone concerned about a future anorectic condition, but it represents a very different issue from whether there is a relationship between risk variables. Relationships are most readily identified by correlational analysis that tells us whether one set of scores relates to another set across a sample of subjects. However, when you are dealing with a low baserate disorder like anorexia nervosa, even on a college campus, co-variation of factors may appear in only a small subset of the sample but still be noteworthy. There may be little overall relationship between two risk variables, but they may still be of joint predictive significance if they converge in the few women who share a serious risk for anorexia nervosa.

As I discussed early in this book, questions regarding whether risk factors actually alter the vulnerability of the woman to eventual anorexia nervosa will not be submitted to clinical proof of actual disorder. Cross-sectional at-risk research cannot identify who within a presumed normal population actually capitulates to this disorder. Longitudinal tracking of the same subjects over an extended time would best accomplish that. However, I chose to fill this void of information when investigating multifactorial risk patterns in much the same way that new risk variables were independently identified in the previous chapter. Just as elevations in stress served to identify new risk factors, increments in stress will be introduced as an indicator of combined risk. If a subset of women demonstrating a full coalition of anorectic risk factors reports more stress than other subsets showing fewer risk indicators (or none), I will conclude that the women showing the full coalition are at more serious anorectic risk. The rationale for this conclusion has been presented more than once, but it bears repeating.

When considering risk at a preliminary stage of anorectic development, excessive stress in a college woman demonstrating early signs of the disorder helps to verify the presence of serious personal problems, most notably problems of competition and achievement. The stress-provoking failures in progressing toward the usual career and social goals make it more likely that the woman will pursue some substitute goal such as a thin body. Stress, or, better said, escape from stress, also serves as a source of motivation for food restraint and for adopting the cognitive mechanisms that assist food restraint. The more stress, the greater the motivation to escape its noxious qualities. Reductions in stress, although temporary and fleeting, strengthen the woman's resolve to lose weight. For other college women who seem to be experiencing the same dissatisfactions by showing elevated anorectic profiles but do not report high levels of stress, there is reason to believe that they do not take these problems seriously. Without serious concern, there is little need for assigning priority to thinness as an alternate goal.

The value of examining patterning effects for the risk variables uncovered by our research goes to the heart of the predictive process for professionals who are likely to come in contact with young-adult women at preclinical stages of stress-related disorder. Concern about anorectic development may grow as the number of observed risk markers increases. It is important to know, given the difficulties inherent in clinical prediction, whether a collection of anorectic risk indicators should be regarded as more pathognomic than some lesser number. Logic says that this should be the case, but if logic always served us well, who would need clinical research?

Studies of Anorectic Risk Patterns Involving Self-preoccupation

I expressed the opinion earlier in this book that if there is a "master trait" underlying stress and anorectic risk, it would be self-preoccupation. The extent to which the person remains acutely aware of herself and interprets the world in terms of differences between herself and others involve elements of both attention and perception. Attention is involved to the extent that the woman focuses predominately upon her own person, her own behavior, and her own fortunes in transacting with the environment. Perception is involved when self-preoccupation leads the woman to selectively interpret experiences in terms of their personal relevance and to slant these personal references toward how she differs from other people.

Being self-preoccupied already has been proposed as critical to anorectic vulnerability as it provides a basis in personality from which other cognitive anorectic risk factors may evolve. Self-preoccupation, then, not only could serve as a specific risk factor for anorexia nervosa in itself but also could contribute to vulnerability by promoting the appearance of other indicators of risk. The importance of an overriding self-preoccupation can be inferred as well from its emergence as an indicator of risk for all three stress-related disorders considered in this book. Besides these arguments for the critical contribution of self-preoccupation as a risk variable, the special role it could play in the theoretical dynamics of anorectic development accentuates its importance even more. I will take a moment to expand upon this view.

Self-preoccupation gains its central position in fomenting the risk of anorexia nervosa because it is capable of assuming a causal role in promoting anomalous forms of cognition and, in turn, being intensified by these emerging cognitive risk factors. Given a continuing exposure to the problems of achievement failure and a reluctance to assume the adult roles that loom ahead, it is little wonder that some young-adult women may become preoccupied with their personal dilemmas and subject to excessive stress. This self-preoccupation may destine the choice of bodily thinness as a substitute goal, since her acute awareness of the self would make selection of a goal integral to her person more likely. Once that the body is assigned such priority, only adding to her self-preoccupation, the woman's inclination to direct her attention and slant her perceptions toward herself would provide fertile psychological ground for the cognitive distortions that add to the risk of overly-successful dieting. Distortions of body image and the continuous concern about food restraint and body changes that goes into serious dieting should add to the woman's awareness of herself as should her monitoring of the physical differences between herself and others, particularly other women. Self-preoccupation gathers strength from the cognitive changes that it has helped to generate. This cause-and-effect role is what makes self-preoccupation such an important source of anorectic vulnerability by my analysis.

Sex-role status and self-preoccupation as combined anorectic risk factors. College women who were themselves feminine or who were sensitive to traditional sex-role differences were found more at-risk for anorexia nervosa (Heilbrun & Mulqueen, 1987; Heilbrun & Putter, 1986); so, too, were self-preoccupied women (Heilbrun & Flodin, 1989). Gender-role appears important as a source of risk for much the same reason as self-preoccupation. This complex role variable contributes several behavioral dispositions that augment the risk of anorexia nervosa as I have proposed its origins in college women. For one thing, the more traditional female is less well-equipped psychologically for competition because of her expressive orientation and commitment to interpersonal harmony. Reluctance in competition has been proposed as a source of goal-oriented failure and stress and, in turn, greater self-preoccupation in the feminine woman. In addition, femi-

nine college women have been reported as more keenly invested in a
thin body, beyond even the pervasive standard of thinness that is found
in our society. Priority given to a thin body by the feminine and/or
role-sensitive woman readily translates into selection as a substitute
goal and into dieting and body-preoccupation should she elect to
switch her priorities.

Since a relationship is thought to exist between femininity and self-
preoccupation, some empirical documentation regarding their mutual
roles within an anorectic risk pattern is needed. The question remains
whether the gender-role and self-preoccupation variables introduce
some degree of risk independently of the other so that the college
woman who is both feminine and self-preoccupied is at greater anorectic risk than the woman who displays one characteristic but not the
other (or neither). Following the procedures of at-risk analysis, the
question actually becomes whether high stress as a fourth risk factor is
unique to women who display the other three indicators of risk -- high
AP status, a feminine identity, and high self-preoccupation. Stress will
serve not only as a risk factor in itself but as a marker of importance for
the entire pattern in projecting anorectic vulnerability.

Heilbrun, Frank, and Friedberg (1991) gathered a broad array of
data that, among other things, allowed them to consider the coalescence
of femininity and self-preoccupation in high AP college women and
their combined effect upon anorectic risk. The battery of psychological
measures in this study included some with which the reader is familiar
(EDI, stress symptoms), but two others require a word of explanation.
The measurement of sex-role orientation was based upon the Adjective
Check List (Gough & Heilbrun, 1965; 1980) using independent Femininity and Masculinity scales developed by Heilbrun (1976). Providing
separate femininity and masculinity scores was in keeping with con-
sensual measurement procedures that have been in place since the
1970s. Sex-role researchers agreed that these dispositions develop
independently, so that the development of one type of sex-role behavior
does not preclude the development of the other. Sex-role make-up,
then, is most aptly described in terms of the relative strength of both
dispositions. Heilbrun, Frank, and Friedberg assigned standard scores
($M = 50$, $SD = 10$) to each scale based upon female college norms.
They then defined feminine women as those who provided feminine
scores in excess of their masculine scores; women showing the opposite
pattern were considered masculine.

The second commentary on measurement involves the self-preoccupation variable. Research reported earlier included self-ratings on perceived effects of food in which the subject reported her sense of body changes when eating was anticipated or had been completed. These perceived experiences were used to gauge the woman's sensitivity to her body and were presented as an aspect of bodily self-preoccupation. A more rigorous and generalized measure of self-preoccupation was available to us by the time of the 1991 Heilbrun, Frank, and Friedberg study, tested for utility in earlier studies within the stress research programs (Heilbrun & Frank, 1989; Heilbrun & Friedberg, 1987; Heilbrun & Hausman, 1990). The idea underlying this more general measure of self-preoccupation involved mental networks that become organized around particular categories of information -- cognitive schemas. The reader may remember that we used schema measurement in previous research as a basis for estimating the woman's sensitivity to traditional sex-role assignments. Many years before that, researchers found evidence for the self-schema that includes information relevant to the self (Bransford & Franks, 1971; Markus, 1977). They concluded that a strong self-schema would lead the person to be acutely aware of herself, to view the world in terms of differences between herself and others, and to better remember information if it pertained to herself. A well-developed self-schema in a research sense is equivalent in meaning to self-preoccupation as I have used the term.

We developed our own version of a self-schema measurement procedure, assisted greatly by earlier innovative work in the Emory laboratory by Madison (1983). The procedure involved three tasks, administered in two laboratory sessions separated by about a week. This complicated procedure is described in detail within all of the papers published by Heilbrun and his co-workers cited previously (Heilbrun & Frank, 1989; Heilbrun & Friedberg, 1989; Heilbrun & Hausman, 1990). Only its essential features will be described here. In the first laboratory session, the woman was asked to describe herself on a 300-item checklist of behavioral adjectives. In the week between sessions, each subject had test materials prepared especially for her based upon her self-description. When the subject returned a week later, she was presented an 80-item checklist, half self-descriptive and half not. She was asked to review this list with respect to self-descriptiveness; this instruction was simply a device to expose her to the items that were and were not self-relevant. Ten minutes after reviewing this list and without prior warning, the woman was given a final checklist of 80 adjectives that included 40 from the recently reviewed list (20 self-descriptive and 20 not) and another 40 from the larger list seen a week before but not in this session (20 self-relevant and 20 not). The subject rated each trait regarding whether it was present on the list seen 10 minutes before using scales representing degree of certainty.

The self-schema score was based upon a multiple-term memory formula that compared the certainty of recall for self-relevant items actually on the list viewed 10 minutes earlier with the certainty accorded to items on that list that were not self-characteristic (i.e., a true-positive effect). The formula also included a false-positive effect, the difference in memory confidence for self-relevant items not on the list from 10 minutes earlier compared to items not on the list and not self-relevant. The way that the formula was scored, higher scores indicated a more vivid memory for self-descriptive traits whether the woman is correct in her recollection or not. This kind of effect in which all terms relevant to the self are more vividly remembered would mark a stronger self-schema and denote greater self-preoccupation.

Before considering the critical question of risk coalescence involving stress as the barometer of combined risk, the prior question of coincidence in a correlational sense was analyzed. Do femininity and self-preoccupation tend to coincide within a high AP group of women? The 55 college women in the study were first split into high and low AP scores at the sample median. Gender-role was defined by subtracting the Masculinity scale score from the Femininity score, with plus scores identifying feminine women. Self-preoccupation scores received a median split. When high AP subjects were examined, 80% of those who were more self-preoccupied also qualified as more feminine. In contrast, only 43% of the more self-preoccupied women in the low AP group qualified as feminine ($p < .05$). Femininity and self-preoccupation as risk factors tend to co-exist in women symptomatically at-risk for anorectic development.

Does the femininity/high self-preoccupation pattern portend greater anorectic risk as evidenced by high stress levels? This question was addressed by comparing the stress scores for 11 women presumably at greatest risk within the sample (high AP, feminine, and high self-preoccupation) with two other less vulnerable groups. Those at moderate risk included 11 high AP women who showed either femininity or high self-preoccupation but not both. The 33 low-risk women either displayed high AP scores without further indication of risk or low AP scores without regard to additional risk factors. Stress scores across these groups were: Greatest risk, $\underline{M}$ = 59.55; moderate risk, $\underline{M}$ = 43.64; low risk, $\underline{M}$ = 34.30. The stark differences in stress along with statistical verification of significant variation ($\underline{p}$ < .001) provide clearcut evidence for a risk pattern involving both gender-role and self-preoccupation. Women who present preclinical anorectic symptoms, a feminine sex-role orientation, and are more self-preoccupied also show the fourth risk factor, an excessive level of stress. This pattern of four risk factors suggests a compounded vulnerability to eventual anorexia nervosa.

The influence of food cues upon perceived body size and self-preoccupation. When the introduction of food cues tends to expand the perceived body size of photographed women models for high AP females, anorectic risk increases. Replicated evidence showed that body-enhancers with an elevated anorectic profile reported a heavy burden of stress. When this perceptual mechanism was studied in terms of the personal eating experiences of female subjects, a similar phenomenon was observed for the high AP woman. Those who experienced a sense of an expanded body in the face of actual food cues reported the most stress related to eating and also endorsed a number of other idiosyncrasies characteristic of the serious dieter. This perceptual mechanism in which food cues elicit enhanced body size was readily conceptualized as a strategy of food restraint. It was proposed to be an aspect of self-preoccupation as well, in this case a preoccupation with one's own body.

Heilbrun and Hausman (1990) used 56 college women to consider the questions regarding coalescence for perceived increase in body size induced by food cues and high self-preoccupation within a high AP group. Do they tend to be associated in a high AP group and does their common presence result in an increment of risk? Procedures in this investigation involved presentation of the EDI and the stress measure to the subjects before exposing them individually to the laboratory procedures. Both laboratory tasks have been described on previous pages. One was concerned with the effect of food cues upon perceived body-size of photographed models, and the other considered self-schema as an indicator of self-preoccupation.

The preliminary question of whether bodies being perceived as larger in response to food cues is associated with greater self-preoccupation in the high AP female can be answered by reference to Table 5.1. It can be seen that the highest level of self-preoccupation

Table 5.1.   Self-preoccupation in High and Low AP College Women, Further Subdivided by Presence or Absence of Perceptual Body Enhancement in the Presence of Food Cues

Perceptual Effect	More Anorectic Characteristics		Fewer Anorectic Characteristics	
	N	M	N	M
Body Enhancement	16	43.12	14	32.29
Body Nonenhancement	12	14.33	14	35.40

Note. - Adapted from Heilbrun, A. B., & Hausman, G. A. (1990). Perceived enhancement of body size in women sharing anorexic psychological characteristics: The role of self-preoccupation. International Journal of Eating Disorders, 9, 283-291.

was found for those high AP females who also displayed body enhancement with food cues present ($\underline{M}$ = 43.12). Equally striking, women with more anorectic symptoms who lacked this body-enhancing perceptual mechanism presented an extremely low level of self-preoccupation ($\underline{M}$ = 14.33). These two extremes of self-preoccupation within the high AP group differed from each other statistically ($\underline{p}$ < .05). Control women split into enhancers and nonenhancers showed intermediate levels of self-preoccupation that varied little from each other.

These results suggest that women who are at some symptomatic risk for anorectic development to begin with and who also show the body-enhancement mechanism are highly preoccupied with themselves. The high AP woman who for whatever reason has not fallen heir to this cognitive source of food restraint demonstrates a low level of self-preoccupation. Said another way, high AP women tend to show both risk factors or show neither. Control females displayed no association between the two cognitive traits.

Why high AP women gravitate toward the extremes of self-preoccupation, depending upon whether they show the perceptual mechanism or not, remains a matter for conjecture. My personal hunch, in the absence of evidence, is that it has to do with how seriously the young-adult female takes the problematic development associated with anorectic risk. If she can deal with her achievement dilemma with equanimity (without much self-preoccupation), body thinness as a substitute goal would take on less significance. Perceptual distortion of the body when exposed to food cues, in turn, would prove unnecessary. If the woman is more responsive to her problems and is more self-preoccupied, her chances of shifting greater priority to body thinness are increased. The perceptual mechanism is activated as food restraint becomes more central to her life. Self-preoccupation comes first; body preoccupation follows.

The sample of women was divided into three groups in order to determine whether the perceptual mechanism inflating body-size and self-preoccupation operate independently as risk factors. Stress once again served as the barometer of risk. A high-risk group (assuming independent contributions) included high AP subjects who also were body-enhancers and who fell above the sample median on self-preoccupation. An intermediate-risk group included all other high AP women whether they showed one risk factor or neither, and the low-risk group was made up of low-AP females without regard to the risk factors.Table 5.2 reports the average level of daily stress for these groups.

Statistical examination of the three stress means reported in Table 5.2 revealed an overall significant variation ($p < .001$). Direct comparison of the high risk group with the intermediate-risk high AP females ($p < .05$) and the low-risk control women ($p < .001$) confirmed the especially high level of stress reported by high AP women showing both specific risk factors. Perceptual body enhancement and self-preoccupation combine in the high AP female to increase anorectic risk as shown by high stress scores, so they do seem to make independent contributions to vulnerability within this four-factor anorectic risk pattern.

The procedure we used for grouping our subjects in this risk analysis appears to favor achieving the outcome we did. The intermediate-risk group includes high AP women who show one specific risk-conferring factor but not the other. However, these are combined with high AP subjects showing neither specific risk factor. Since the latter set of women should be relatively free of stress, there might be concern that the low stress reported by the high AP women demonstrating neither specific risk factor might mask the elevated stress experienced by high AP women who did display one or the other. This was not the case. High AP women characterized by either the perceptual mechanism or self-preoccupation actually revealed a slightly lower stress score ($M = 44.30$) than the high AP women characterized by neither ($M = 45.81$). The full complement of risk indicators was required before peak stress levels were confirmed.

Studies of Anorectic Risk Patterns Involving Factors from the Same and Different Cognitive Categories

Earlier in the book I presented a convenient way of categorizing the various cognitive functions in terms of how the individual deals with stimulation that continuously presents itself from within or from our external environment. Deployment of attention determines the source of stimulation upon which we focus. Perception represents the meaning we assign to that stimulation. Processing refers to how we deal with meaningful stimulation (information). Each cognitive category requires further breakdown into numerous specific functions. To this point we have considered attention in terms of degree of sensitivity to focal stimulation (e.g., the disattention mechanisms in bulimic and anorectic risk). Perception has been treated in terms of need-responsive function

Table 5.2.   Stress Reported by High AP Women Displaying Body
Enhancement and High Self-preoccupation, All Other High
AP Women, and Controls

High AP Women Displaying Body Enhancement and High Self-preoccupation		All Other High AP Women		All Control Women	
N	M	N	M	N	M
11	56.18	17	44.52	28	32.36

Note. - Adapted from Heilbrun, A. B., & Hausman, G. A.
(1990). Perceived enhancement of body size in women sharing
anorexic psychological characteristics: The role of self-preoccupation.
International Journal of Eating Disorders, 9, 283-291.

in which meaning assigned to stimulation serves a convenient motivational purpose (e.g., body-imaging and body-enhancement mechanisms). Processing was at issue when the woman's strategy of defense against threatening information was examined (e.g., repression and other mechanisms of defense).

Specific risk factors from different cognitive categories. One set of questions that remained toward the end of the anorectic research program concerned the relationship between risk variables that find representation within different or the same cognitive categories. This issue bears upon whether risk of anorexia nervosa in the individual case is contingent upon the vulnerability of a particular cognitive category to distortion of information or whether cognition tends to be compromised across categories. An answer to this question would assist professional intervention to the extent that the search for risk factors could be concentrated within one cognitive category or spread more broadly if it were known whether at-risk women are betrayed by a wider band of cognitive functions. The evidence on specific risk factors in the previous two chapters suggested that attention, perception, and processing variables can be implicated. However, we did not collect this evidence in such a way as to address the present issue in a definitive way -- by examining cognitive risk variables from different categories as they are represented in the same women. Heilbrun and Lozman (1991) conducted a study that considered whether cognitive deficit tends to be restricted to one category in promoting anorectic risk or can be expected to spread across categories in the individual case.

Heilbrun and Lozman sampled 75 college women in their investigation of perception/attention patterning effects. Perceived body image and disattention to the sensations of hunger were chosen for study. They represented different cognitive categories, each had been independently confirmed as a specific risk variable, and that both would contribute to food restraint for the high AP woman seemed obvious. The actual evidence reported on earlier pages included the replicated finding that women with high anorectic profiles had distorted body images but only if they were on the thin side (Heilbrun & Friedberg, 1990, 1991; Heilbrun & Witt, 1990). Disattention to internal sensations of hunger was found to be associated with anorectic risk (Heilbrun & Worobow, 1990) and was an especially striking result in light of other findings that the at-risk female was not insensitive to other internal sensations associated with hunger -- those signaling hunger satiety

(Heilbrun & Worobow, 1991).

Although 75 subjects usually qualified as sufficient for studying the research questions in our program, it proved to be a marginal number in this case, because we drew a skewed sample as far as AP scores were concerned. By this I mean that the 75 women included far more with lower AP scores than had been true in prior studies. I doubt if this represented some kind of trend on campus; more than likely, it was a random sampling effect. In any case, AP scores had to be divided at three points rather than the usual division at the mid-point in order to identify a "high AP" group that matched the scores of previous samples. While the upper third of the EDI profile scores provided a high AP grouping comparable to the high categories of other at-risk studies, intermediate (middle third) and low (lower third) AP groups obtained scores that would have been in the low AP range before. This sampling effect had to be taken into consideration as I examined the stress results.

Both the perceptual and attentional mechanisms under investigation by Heilbrun and Lozman were complex effects dependent on two components. The approach we used to measure these complex risk variables was to combine the two scores contributing to each into a single index. This allowed us to keep the logistical demands of the investigation within manageable limits by conserving on the subjects required for analysis. In order to obtain the perceptual index of risk, the subject's body-size and body-image scores, obtained as before, were each transformed into the same standard-score distribution with a mean of 50 (standard deviation of 10). Lower body size and higher BPI scores were assigned higher standard score equivalents, because it was the thinner woman who was most prone to distorting her body image. By multiplying the two scores for each subject, we can estimate how closely the high AP woman approximates this risk prototype by showing a thinner body and inflated body image. The same procedure was used to provide an index of attentional risk. Scores were combined on two TAIS scales -- Reduced Attentional Focus and Overload of Internal Stimulation. Higher scores on these scales allow for the insensitivity and inner tumult that would make it easier for the high AP woman to ignore hunger sensations. A higher multiplicative score reflects the potential for the disattentional mechanism underlying food restraint.

Table 5.3 includes mean disattention values for the sample of women broken down by three AP levels and by high and low perceptual distortion of body image based upon a median split of the sample distribution. The overall statistical effect was a triple interaction ($p < .05$)

Table 5.3.   Disattention to Inner Sensations for College Women Separated by Anorectic Profile and Body-image Distortion

| High Anorectic Profile | | | | Intermediate Anorectic Profile | | | | Low Anorectic Profile | | | |
| Presence of Body-image Distortion | | Absence of Body-image Distortion | | Presence of Body-image Distortion | | Absence of Body-image Distortion | | Presence of Body-image Distortion | | Absence of Body-image Distortion | |
N	M	N	M	N	M	N	M	N[a]	M	N	M
12	3215.42	14	2643.78	9	2383.78	15	2149.93	17	2241.18	8	2781.88

[a] The substantial number of low AP women included in this "presence of body-image distortion" group resulted from their very thin body sizes and not from inflated image.

Note. - Adapted from Heilbrun, A. B., & Lozman, R. (1991). Body-image distortion and disattention to internal stimulation: Alternative or common anorectic risk factors. Currently unpublished study.

brought about by an effect found at one AP extreme reversing itself at the other extreme. Women who were at-risk because of high AP scores and because they were thin and perceptually distorted their body images also obtained singularly high disattention scores. The two specific anorectic risk variables, one perceptual and the other attentional, did coalesce within the set of women already at-risk because of their anorectic profiles. The intermediate AP group findings revealed no relationship between the risk variables; rather similar disattention scores were registered whether the women displayed the body-image/body-size risk factor or not. By the time you reach the low AP group, you can see that the disattention scores have reversed themselves when comparing body-image/body-size subgroups. Women who show body-image distortion and a thinner body show considerably less potential for disattention.

These results present clearcut evidence of a patterning effect across cognitive categories. Perceptual and attentional food-restraining mechanisms appear together in females already at symptomatic risk for anorexia nervosa, the association disappears as AP status decreases, and the two risk variables become mutually exclusive in low AP women.

Stress was analyzed next in order to go beyond the question of coalescence to whether the combined presence of the perceptual and attentional mechanisms augments anorectic risk in the high AP woman. Examination failed to reveal increased stress to be associated with a pattern involving high AP status, body-image distortion -- both defined as before -- and heightened disattention given by scores above the sample median. High AP women demonstrating both risk factors had much the same level of stress as high AP women who displayed only one or the other. Thus, the most difficult discrimination required to verify a coalescence effect of anorectic risk factors upon reported stress failed to materialize.

Although we were unable to find a cumulative stress effect across the entire risk pattern, there was evidence that stress remained part of the risk picture. The 21 college women with high anorectic profiles and who displayed one or both additional markers of vulnerability reported stress scores averaging 52.52. The 36 remaining women in the sample (intermediate and low AP) giving evidence of these cognitive mechanisms provided far lower average scores of 41.72 ($\underline{p} < .01$). Thus, distortions of perception and attention, alone or in combination, signal anorectic risk but only if the woman is also beginning to display other anorectic characteristics. However, if neither cognitive mechanism is apparent, there is little difference in stress between high AP females ($\underline{M}$ = 34.00, $\underline{N}$ = 5) and those at the intermediate and low AP levels ($\underline{M}$ = 31.32, $\underline{N}$ = 13).

Although I remain uncertain about how to explain the limited augmentation of risk within the pattern studied by Heilbrun and Lozman, the results have to stand for the time being. High AP women who either demonstrated body-image distortion or who were found capable of disattention to inner sensations of hunger reported as much stress as those high AP females who displayed both cognitive mechanisms. The unusual distribution of AP scores could have somehow put a cap on extreme stress scores or introduced other unrepresentative effects, but I have no evidence that this is true.

Heilbrun and Lozman did an additional analysis of the risk patterning effects for our female subjects in which body size (i.e., the weight/height ratio) was taken into consideration independently of body image rather than being combined in a single index with it. Body thinness had been identified as a contributing risk factor within the body-image studies when distortion was found primarily in thin women. This implies that heavier women are in little danger of becoming anorectic, because they would be less likely to use this food-restraining perceptual mechanism. Perhaps actual body size might serve as a motivation for dieting, but their body images would be counterproductive in that they underrepresented their actual size. It remained possible though that larger women, at least those with a high AP profile, come to depend upon a disattentional strategy of food restraint even if body-image distortion is unlikely. Since present results suggest that the presence of one can promote as much anorectic risk as both, heavier women could turn out to be more vulnerable than it might otherwise seem.

We divided each of our three AP levels into three body sizes according to whether the woman's weight/height ratio qualified her as thinnest third, average, or fattest third for the sample. The body-imaging scores, examined independently for these nine groups using the BPI, showed exactly what we found in the previous studies for high AP women; an expanded body image was commonplace in the thinnest third, an unrealistically slimmer body image was observed at the heaviest extreme, and those of average bodies provided realistic body images ($\underline{p}$ < .01). Only the thinnest among high AP women showed a distorted body image, the third time that a coalition between a thin body, perceptual distortion, and preclinical anorectic symptoms had been demonstrated in our research program. As before, women without high anorectic profiles revealed similar body-imaging scores suggesting underestimation.

When disattention scores of high AP women were considered, we found that those at both the thinnest and fattest extremes of body size showed clearcut potential for disattention to internal sensations, and the mechanism was absent in those of average weight ($p < .05$). Intermediate and low AP women, broken down by body size, presented no differences in level of disattention.

I conclude from this rather complicated alignment of body size, body image, and disattention in the Heilbrun and Lozman data that thinner women are still more at-risk given a high anorectic profile. However, high AP women at the other body extreme are more vulnerable than I believed when the earlier body-image studies were conducted. Thinner females with high anorectic profiles are almost certain to possess one cognitive mechanism or the other, likely both, to assist in food restraint. Fatter high AP women are not going to invoke body-image distortion to motivate dieting but many of them will be capable of disregarding hunger sensations. These heaviest of high AP women in our sample are not free of increments in anorectic risk promoted by cognitive mechanisms conducive to food restraint. They do appear to be less likely to possess such a mechanism, however, when compared to their thin high AP counterparts who show both perceptual distortion and disattention.

Testing the limits of the at-risk method -- a six-factor risk pattern for anorexia nervosa. The Heilbrun and Friedberg (1991) study was viewed as the last opportunity to tie loose ends together concerning risk factors for anorexia nervosa before assembling the evidence for the present book. This omnibus investigation considered several items, although the most important among these had to do with whether we should expect increments in risk, defined by increasing stress, as more and more factors appear in the risk pattern. Heilbrun and Lozman (1991), in a study I have just reviewed, found that risk did not seem to escalate when high AP women displayed both body-image distortion and the potential for disattention to hunger sensations relative to the presence of either cognitive mechanism alone. If either mechanism (or both) were in evidence, however, the high AP female did show more stress than if she were free of cognitive distortion, although it was rare to find high-profile women without a distended body image or selective attention.

I found the logic of incremental risk with added markers of vulnerability to be too compelling to let the matter rest. Accordingly, the importance of extended risk patterns was a paramount concern for Heilbrun and Friedberg as we examined a different combination of factors. Given that we were able to demonstrate a trend toward increasing stress as broader risk patterns were examined, a related question would be addressed. How far could we carry the compiling of risk factors while still requiring that added stress must accompany increments in pattern size? We ended up attempting a six-factor pattern of anorectic vulnerability.

Other residual issues also were investigated. For one, body-image distortion and body enhancement in response to food cues are similar-sounding perceptual mechanisms serving food restraint. Are they independent risk factors, or are they simply different ways of measuring the same thing? For another, the psychological defenses represent cognitive-processing variables that have been related to anorectic risk; do these processing variables contribute to risk independently of the cognitively distinct perceptual variables. The prior effort to demonstrated an independent contribution to risk across perceptual and attentional cognitive categories was unsuccessful, as you know.

Heilbrun and Friedberg investigated body enhancement in the presence of food cues (using laboratory procedures), body image, psychological defense, anorectic profiles, actual body size, and stress symptoms using standard measurement procedures that have been described in earlier studies. Only the scoring of defenses departs from the original and requires a brief recapitulation of the earlier results. At-risk women preferred a repressive defense that involved selective forgetting of distressing information. This result received major emphasis for two reasons. A repressive defense offered the dynamics most conducive to poor problem resolution and helped to explain the failure to resolve the achievement dilemma. It also had been found to be associated with the greatest stress in other studies. However, a second significant finding found at-risk women to be less inclined to use projection as a defense, a strategy which involved the assignment of unfavorable traits to others to improve one's own self-image. Psychological analysis of these two defenses suggests that repression is a totally self-contained cognitive operation, not dependent upon external events or people. Projection, in contrast, involves a marked sensitivity to external events and people as the person seeks relief from personal liabilities by perceptually altering the social environment. Since later research emphasized the self-preoccupation of the woman at anorectic risk, this pattern of defense (i.e., high repression/low-projection) attracts the following explanation. Self-preoccupation of at-risk women may lead them to gravitate toward a self-contained defense and away from a defense requiring sensitivity to others and fixing upon external events. It is a high repression/low projection defense pattern that best conforms to the insular dictates of self-preoccupation.

This repression/projection pattern, rather than repression alone, contributes to the woman's failure to resolve her achievement problems in two ways. It not only involves a maximum distancing from awareness for her problems (high repression), but it allows her to remain displaced psychologically from the social environment (low projection) within which her on-going troubles in competing for career and social goals are vested. The seeming importance of both defenses as risk factors was captured in an index based upon the difference between repression and projection scores. A plus difference would denote a self-contained and isolating pattern of defense, poorer resolution of socially-based problems, and anorectic risk. A negative difference should be reserved for someone more attuned to the social environment, less self-preoccupied, and at lower risk for anorexia nervosa.

Given the experience with Heilbrun and Lozman's (1991) multi-factorial study in which a skewed distribution of AP scores required a tripartite separation to reveal curvilinear relationships, the present investigation collected a larger sample ($\underline{N}$ = 100) of college women with an eye to using the same three-level division. Our first analysis focused upon the two body-perception factors and the issue of their independence. Table 5.4 summarizes the BPI body-image scores for women assigned by AP level and whether they were body enhancers or nonenhancers when food cues were introduced along with the photographs of models in the laboratory procedure. The most general statistical test revealed no overall relationship between body imaging and body enhancement represented in these average figures. The fact that the 55 enhancers had about the same body-image score ($\underline{M}$ = 103.76) as the 45 nonenhancers ($\underline{M}$ = 101.76) and that the scores were not related across the entire sample puts to rest any concern about their representing essentially equivalent forms of body perception.

The one significant finding that was identified by our statistics was embedded within the array of scores reported in Table 5.4. If only one

Table 5.4. Body-image Distortion for College Women Differing in Anorectic Characteristics and Body Enhancement in the Presence of Food Cues

	Anorectic Characteristics					
	High		Intermediate		Low	
Body Perception with Food Cues	N	M	N	M	N	M
Enhancement	20	112.45	20	98.45	15	99.27
Nonenhancement	11	100.09	15	104.87	19	100.26

Note. - From Heilbrun, A. B., & Friedberg, L. (1991). Elaboration of a proposed cognitive network underlying the development of anorexia nervosa. Currently unpublished study.

effect were to be found, however, none would present the critical argument for coalescence of perceptual risk factors as turned out to be the case. Considering high AP women only, those who enhanced female body size when food cues were introduced also maintained a distorted body image ($\underline{M}$ = 112.45). Women with comparable AP scores but who lacked the body-enhancing mechanism offered no sign of body-image distortion ($\underline{M}$ = 100.09). This difference was reliable ($\underline{p}$ < .05). For female subjects most at-risk based on their symptomatic similarity to anorectics, the presence of perceptual mechanisms geared to food restraint tended to be all-or-nothing. Roughly two-thirds of the high AP women were body enhancers in response to food stimulation, and these women also distorted their body images when food cues were not present. Anorectic vulnerability may well escalate in these cases because of the presence of all three risk factors. The one-third of the high-AP group (along with the remaining women in the sample) who were lacking in paired mechanisms would be less at-risk.

The next analysis considered the defense-index scores for the same six groups that figured in the previous table -- three levels of AP scores subdivided into those who did and did not enhance body size in the presence of food cues. Table 5.5 includes the defense findings, and statistics confirm a general AP effect ($\underline{p}$ < .05) as well as an AP x body-enhancement interaction ($\underline{p}$ < .001). The origin of both effects can be traced to the defense scores for high AP females which are vastly out of line with those found in the remainder of the table. At this extreme level of AP, a relatively strong preference for self-contained repression over socially-sensitive projection is apparent among enhancers ($\underline{M}$ = 9.35), and the opposite preference for projection over repression stands out for nonenhancers ($\underline{M}$ = -9.00). These divergent patterns of psychological defense differ significantly ($\underline{p}$ < .001). Body enhancers and nonenhancers at the lower two AP levels were very similar in their defense scores and noncommittal as groups regarding a preference for repression or projection.

Coalescence of specific risk factors was observed, then, at the high AP level where women who responded to food cues by perceptually enhancing body size also favored a more self-contained style of defense. The association is presumably fostered by a common relationship to self-preoccupation. In contrast, a socially-oriented defense is used by high AP nonenhancers, made possible by the absence of self-preoccupation. This linkage between perception and cognitive-processing variables, which may serve to escalate risk in high AP

Table 5.5. Pattern of Defense[a] for College Women Differing in Anorectic Characteristics and Body Enhancement in the Presence of Food Cues

| | Anorectic Characteristics | | | | | |
| | High | | Intermediate | | Low | |
Body Perception with Food Cues	N	M	N	M	N	M
Enhancement	20	9.35	20	-2.24	15	2.20
Nonenhancement	11	-9.00	15	1.75	19	2.29

[a]Plus scores indicate a defensive style favoring self-contained repression over socially-sensitive projection, and minus scores indicate the opposite.

Note. - From Heilbrun, A. B., Friedberg, L. (1991). Elaboration of a proposed cognitive network underlying the development of anorexia nervosa. Currently unpublished study.

women, was not observed in females without high AP scores.

The defense index and body image were next considered together to round out the analysis of defensive processing and perceptual mechanisms across AP levels. Table 5.6 offers the average defense-pattern scores for groups broken down by three AP levels and two body-imaging BPI levels. Body-distortion scores on each side of 100 defined unrealistic degrees of fatness and unrealistic degrees of thinness in keeping with BPI assumptions. No overall effects were obtained for the Table 5.6 means, but, as was true for the analysis involving food-cue-induced body enhancement, an isolated effect was found among the high AP subjects. Those who distorted their body image so as to appear unrealistically fat preferred a repressive defense ($\underline{M}$ = 6.57), whereas the high AP females who imagined themselves to be unrealistically thin showed a slight preference for projection ($\underline{M}$ = -1.88). This difference was reliable ($\underline{p}$ < .05), but nothing came from the same comparison at the remaining two AP levels. The Heilbrun and Friedberg (1991) results to this point suggest that defensive processing and each of the two body-perception variables vary independently of each other over an entire sample of college women. However, they show an all-or-nothing relationship to each other if only high AP women are concerned. Either the three risk factors emerge as a pattern or none appear. Whether this coalescence contributes to added risk will be considered next.

The successive analyses have isolated the three specific risk factors (body enhancement, body image, and a preference for repression over projection) within a subset of females already showing evidence of vulnerability in high AP scores. Given this assembly of risk indicators, it was a matter of special interest to determine whether they would then contribute as a pattern to the developmental risk for anorexia within this high AP group. Despite starting with a substantial number of subjects ($\underline{N}$ = 100), it became necessary to introduce analysis procedures for the four risk factors that would conserve on required subject numbers. The fifth marker of anorectic vulnerability, stress, again would serve as the gauge of risk.

In order to determine whether the defensive processing and perceptual risk factors were associated with escalated stress among high AP women, it first was necessary to establish a pattern score that would reflect the extent to which a subject was characterized by these three cognitive risk variables. Each of the cognitive score distributions was cut into thirds for the entire sample. Points were assigned for each variable depending upon the degree to which the subject demonstrated body

Table 5.6   Pattern of Defense Scores[a] for College Women Differing in Anorectic Characteristics and Body-image Distortion[b]

Body-image Distortion	High		Intermediate		Low	
	$\underline{N}$	$\underline{M}$	$\underline{N}$	$\underline{M}$	$\underline{N}$	$\underline{M}$
Perceived Self as Fatter than Actually is	17	6.57	16	-.12	14	3.50
Perceived Self as Thinner than Actually is	14	-1.88	19	-.58	20	1.55

Anorectic Characteristics

[a]Plus scores indicate a defensive style favoring self-contained repression over socially-sensitive projection, and minus scores suggest the opposite.

[b]Based upon the Body Perception Index.

Note. - From Heilbrun, A. B., & Friedberg, L. (1991). Elaboration of a proposed cognitive network underlying the development of anorexia nervosa. Currently unpublished study.

enhancement in the context of food cues, an unrealistically fat body image, or a repressive (rather than projective) defense. The scoring system involved the following rules: upper third (in the direction of risk) = 3, middle third = 2, lower third = 1. The risk-pattern score for each subject was the sum of these three discrete risk scores. The risk-pattern score, in turn, was divided at its median so that higher-risk (pattern present) and lower-risk (pattern absent) groups could be identified at each of the three AP levels. Stress scores derived from the stress-symptom measure are reported in Table 5.7 for the six AP x risk-pattern subgroups.

One overall statistical effect was evident in the Table 5.7 mean figures; the higher the anorectic profile revealed by the subject, the greater the stress ($p < .01$). Higher levels of stress were confirmed for the high and intermediate AP groups relative to the low AP group. As you examine the stress figures one AP level at a time, a pattern present/absent effect is evident only for high AP women. Those with the cognitive risk pattern present evidenced very strong stress ($M = 59.31$), whereas women with a high anorectic profile but lacking this specific risk pattern reported lower stress ($M = 48.13$), $p < .05$. The intermediate and low AP groups failed to reveal any stress differential between females high and low on the pattern score for cognitive risk factors. Since the 16 women in the sample who revealed evidence of the four anorectic risk indicators also displayed singularly high stress, I would conclude that the accumulation of risk factors adds to anorectic vulnerability.

A distorted body image that conveyed an unrealistic degree of fatness qualified as an important risk factor for high AP women in three earlier studies, but this reliable effect was shown only for those who were thinner in body build. This led me to speculate that an unrealistic perception of herself as overweight would be of special motivational significance in dieting if the woman's thinner proportions contradicted the need for food restraint. Heilbrun and Friedberg took the opportunity to introduce actual body size (weight divided by height) into the analysis of multiple risk factors in order to test the current limits of risk patterns in specifying anorectic vulnerability. Body size was distributed across the sample, cut into three parts, and the following scores assigned: Thinnest third (in the direction of risk) = 3, middle third = 2, fattest third = 1. The body-size score was then added to the woman's sum score for the three cognitive factors to form a four-factor risk-pattern score. As before, the pattern score was cut at its mid-point

Table 5.7.   Stress Reported by College Women Differing in Anorectic
Profile and in the Presence or Absence of a Risk-conferring
Cognitive Pattern[a]

| | Anorectic Profile | | | | | |
| | High | | Intermediate | | Low | |
Presence or Absence of Cognitive Risk Pattern	$\underline{N}$	$\underline{M}$	$\underline{N}$	$\underline{M}$	$\underline{N}$	$\underline{M}$
Pattern Present	16	59.31	13	50.58	11	39.46
Pattern Absent	15	48.13	22	53.62	23	39.39

[a]Including perceived body enhancement in the presence of food cues, perceived body image that is unrealistically heavy, and a preference for repression over projection as a means of defense.

Note. - Heilbrun, A. B., & Friedberg, L. (1991). Elaboration of a proposed cognitive network underlying the development of anorexia nervosa. Currently unpublished study.

to constitute the "presence" or "absence" of the risk-conferring combination.

Table 5.8 summarizes the stress reported for the six groups defined by the three AP levels and the presence or absence of the four-factor risk pattern within each level. The comparison of special interest was within the high AP group. The tendency to present all four specific risk-conferring factors in women symptomatically at-risk for anorexia resulted in an extremely high stress score ($M = 66.20$). The relative absence of these specific factors in high AP subjects was associated with far less stress ($M = 48.05$), $p < .01$. The combined presence of the trio of cognitive risk factors and a thin body was not associated with higher stress at the intermediate or low AP levels. In fact, the very low stress reported by pattern-present, low AP women ($M = 37.56$) testifies to the benign character of the four-factor risk pattern in the absence of a more general anorectic symptom picture.

By narrowing our attention to very high AP females with thinner bodies and the cognitive potential for both problem avoidance and food restraint, we were able to identify college women who are experiencing a level of stress unmatched in any other of our studies on anorectic risk. That level of stress signals the seriousness of the achievement problems facing them as well as the presence of a motivational force driving these women toward relief through a seemingly more attainable accomplishment. The 10 college women who most clearly displayed the six anorectic risk factors represent 10% of the total sample. This begins to approximate the baserate for anorexia nervosa that has been cited on some campuses. This many signs of anorectic risk appearing together in a restricted number of women approaching baserate might mean that the step between vulnerability to disorder and actuality of disorder had been partially bridged by our program of investigation.

Many risk factors identified by our research were not included in the Heilbrun and Friedberg pattern analysis including a direct measure of self-preoccupation, feminine/traditional sex-role commitment, and a body-oriented dieting strategy. Considering this and the rough approximations required for categorical assignment to risk-pattern groups, I am encouraged to believe that we are on the right track toward early detection of anorexia nervosa. Although I cannot specify a rigorous predictive formula for this disorder, that may not be required at this time by health professionals anyway. Knowledge of the factors signaling risk may be enough to alert professionals to the danger of serious psychobiological problems ahead and to offer a direction for interven-

Table 5.8.   Stress Reported by College Women Differing in Anorectic
Profile and the Presence of a Four-factor Risk-conferring
Pattern[a]

Presence or Absence of Risk-conferring Pattern	High		Intermediate		Low	
	N	M	N	M	N	M
Presence	10	66.20	9	54.38	8	37.56
Absence	21	48.05	26	51.92	26	40.04

Anorectic Profile

[a]Including body enhancement in response to food cues, an
unrealistically fat body image, a preference for repression over projection as a defense, and actual body thinness.

Note. - From Heilbrun, A. B., & Friedberg, L. (1991). Elaboration of a proposed cognitive network underlying the development of
anorexia nervosa. Currently unpublished study.

tion. Introducing these factors into an explanatory context of unrequited ambition and a substitute goal of body thinness may offer a further basis for intervening during the risk phase of anorexia nervosa.

Chapter 6

Stress and the Risk of Menstrual Disorder

The contribution of stress and other psychological factors to the risk of serious menstrual disorder in college women will be considered at this time. Restricting the presentation to a single chapter in no way reflects upon the importance of such a risk analysis. It may seem that way when compared with the multiple chapters devoted to understanding anorectic vulnerability already behind us and a similar commitment to detailing the risk of coronary problems in Type As that will follow. The truth of the matter is that there was less evidence I could muster relating to stress and vulnerability to menstrual dysfunction. This did not result from any lack of questions to be put to empirical test or from special difficulties in research method. The stress-and-disorder research program simply ran out of time before there was an opportunity to run the requisite number of studies.

If the research on risk of dysfunctional menstruation is limited compared to our companion studies in anorectic and Type A coronary risk, why even include this evidence in the book? Besides scientific vanity, there is one compelling reason why I did so. It seemed important to consider all of the evidence gathered on risk for stress-related disorders, because doing so allows me to more fully develop the idea that there is a dangerous versatility to stress which allows it to promote psychobiological disorder in a number of ways. To this point, I have emphasized the motivational role of stress in anorectic risk. In broadest terms, I proposed that the woman is diverted from problem-solving and the pursuit of traditional achievement goals to an obsession with thinness and all-too-successful food restraint. Motivational drive for this substitution derives from the aversive nature of stress that energizes and directs behaviors that offer at least short-term escape from distress. Motivational reinforcement from temporary stress reduction strengthens these behaviors, although the source of stress will begin to shift from maturational failures to eating and unwanted fat.

In the chapters ahead I shall have the opportunity to propose a second functional role played by stress in fomenting Type A risk of cardiovascular problems. Stress dynamics in Type A risk cannot be readily understood in terms of motivating the acquisition of behaviors that temporarily reduce stress and are strengthened by stress reduction. In fact, Type A risk factors will be organized in a way that would explain the opposite dynamic; Type As at most serious risk are those who fail to escape from the chronic burden of stress having its origin in an unharnessed need to win and achieve. The functional role attributed to stress in the at-risk Type A is a corrosive one in which the chronic activation of the autonomic nervous system by the emotions of stress eventually takes its toll on the cardiovascular system.

When we examine stress and menstrual dysfunction, the pathogenic role of stress does not appear to be either motivational or as a source of long-term wear-and-tear. Rather, stress seems to operate as an agent of risk by contributing directly to menstrual symptoms in one of two ways. Stress, aroused by developmental problems or by the condition itself, could make menstrual symptoms more severe for her by lowering the woman's tolerance for these aversive changes. Besides increasing her sensitivity, stress could combine its emotional effects with menstrual distress and become part of the worsening symptom pattern. In either case, stress would contribute directly to the discomfort associated with the menstrual cycle and to its disabling qualities.

Perhaps it is more obvious now why the functional role of stress in promoting disorder was said to be dangerously versatile and why it is important to support this thesis by whatever empirical evidence is available. I undertook the investigation of risk for three disorders and came away from each probe by concluding that stress makes its contribution to vulnerability in a different way. How many other psychobiological disorders in women could be linked in yet other ways to the disturbing cognition and emotion of stress, I am not prepared to say. However, if the study of disorder at the preliminary risk stage were continued, it would likely turn up further nuances of stress dynamics.

Menstrual Cycle Dysfunction and Its Measurement

Dysfunction within the menstrual cycle had not as yet been offi-
cially sanctioned as disorder by inclusion in the Diagnostic and Statistical Manual of Mental Disorders at the time I prepared this clinical description. The recent edition, DSM-III-R, does discuss the physical,
emotional, and behavioral changes that begin during the luteal phase of
the cycle when the female body presents the ovum for fertilization and
before the beginning of menstrual flow. If the changes are serious
enough, a provisional diagnosis of "late luteal phase dysphoric disorder" is recommended. The more familiar term, premenstrual
syndrome (PMS), was not favored, but I shall retain PMS to designate
one of the two menstrual disorders for which we sought risk factors.

The diagnostic manual calls to our attention that severe symptoms
may occur within two overlapping periods of the menstrual cycle. The
"late luteal phase" refers to the last week of the luteal phase; the symptoms must begin during this time in order to diagnose PMS. Even
though distressing PMS symptoms begin during the week prior to
menstrual flow, termination of these symptoms may not occur until a
few days after menstruation begins, the follicular phase of the cycle.
The diagnosis of dysmenorrhea (painful menses) is reserved for those
cases in which symptoms appear after the onset of menstrual flow. The
distinction between PMS and dysmenorrhea as clinical disorders, then,
is a matter of timing. These disorders are distinguished by when the
symptoms start and not by the symptoms themselves.

The measurement procedures in this phase of our research, to be
described more fully on the pages ahead, corresponded closely to those
involved in the search for anorectic risk factors. One close parallel
came from the use of the Menstrual Distress Questionnaire (MDQ;
Moos, 1968, 1969, 1986) as a basic indicator of menstrual symptoms at
two vulnerable periods during the menstrual cycle. The Eating Disorders Inventory was used to gauge whether the defining behaviors of
anorexia nervosa were present at a subclinical level in our samples as
well as those central to bulimia. Each questionnaire allowed us to
measure symptoms at an evolving stage when they could serve as evidence of risk rather than providing a litmus test of disorder. There is a
difference in the way that the two psychometric instruments approach
the presentation of symptoms associated with differing forms of disordered eating and disordered menstrual functioning. Eating disorders
are represented by distinct scale combinations. PMS/dysmenorrhea, as
disorders of the menstrual system, are represented by the same symp-

toms. Only their timing distinguishes between indicators of risk for PMS and dysmenorrhea in keeping with psychiatric nosology. Earlier onset of symptoms prior to menstruation is taken as evidence of PMS risk and later onset during menses signals risk of dysmenorrhea.

The diagnoses of PMS or dysmenorrhea are reached when several of the usual changes associated with menstruation reach severe clinical proportions. As I have said, the point in the menstrual cycle when these severe changes make their appearance, before or after the beginning of menstrual flow, determines the specific diagnosis. These symptoms, according to DSM-III-R, include the following:

(1)   unstable emotions
(2)   marked and persistent anger or irritability
(3)   strong anxiety or tension
(4)   seriously depressed mood, feelings of hopelessness, and self-depreciation
(5)   loss of interest in usual activities
(6)   ready fatigue or lack of energy
(7)   difficulty in concentration
(8)   marked change in eating preferences
(9)   oversleeping or insomnia
(10)   physical symptoms including tenderness or swelling of the breast, headaches, pain in the joints or muscles, a sense of bloating, and weight gain.

As is evident, these symptoms would be extremely unpleasant for the woman and will seriously interfere with work, social activities, and just about anything else when the clinical extremes of PMS and dysmenorrhea are reached. What may be less evident is that many of these symptoms correspond to the aversive effects of stress. I will return to this point later in the chapter.

The measurement procedure that we employed for distinguishing degrees of menstrual dysfunction within normal samples of college women involved the use of the Menstrual Distress Questionnaire (MDQ). This is a 47-item self-report inventory that inquires into the physical and psychological changes that are associated with the menstrual cycle. The 47 changes (symptoms) are combined into eight different scales. Seven of these scales contain items that deal with the bad features of menstrual dysfunction and are identified by the test developer as Pain, Concentration, Behavior Change, Autonomic Reaction, Water Retention, Negative Affect, and Control. For the most part, the MDQ items on these seven scales conform reasonably well to the

DSM-III-R list of symptoms for diagnosing menstrual disorder. Only the eighth scale, Arousal (five items), departs radically from the diagnostic manual in that it inquires into more positive feelings associated with menstrual change by some women such as increased feelings of affection, excitement, or well-being. Responses to these five items in my research have usually been out of step with the remainder of the MDQ items that consider negative symptoms; as scores on the 42 negative items have gone up, scores on these five items have dropped. However, a post-hoc check revealed that their inclusion made no difference in the overall MDQ results one way or another (Heilbrun & Frank, 1989). This encouraged me to leave the MDQ as the test developer intended by allowing all questionnaire items to contribute to the final results.

Completing the MDQ requires the subject to rate the severity of each of the 47 symptoms on six-point scales extending from "no experience of symptom" (score = 1) on the low end to "acute or partially disabling" (score = 6) on the higher severity end. The previously completed menstrual cycle is used as the basis for these ratings; Moos confirmed that this procedure was a satisfactory substitute for ratings based upon several cycles. Actually, the woman is asked to make three successive ratings over the same set of 47 symptoms. She records symptom severity for the menstrual (flow) period, the premenstrual (week before flow) span,and the intermenstrual (remainder of cycle) interval. Scoring for the MDQ in our studies ignored the assignment of symptoms to the eight scales, since our analyses were directed at general malaise rather than discrete categories of symptoms. Instead, we combined the woman's ratings on all 47 items into a single composite distress score. The scoring procedure was repeated for each of the three time-defined rating sets giving us an overall premenstrual, menstrual, and intermenstrual distress score.

Logue and Moos (1986) have recommended that MDQ symptom scores be determined relative to a baseline of complaint for each subject. This procedure would accomplish two things. They emphasize the benefit of controlling styles of reporting personal distress. Some individuals may describe menstrual experience in more vivid terms than others even though the intensity of the changes is much the same. Determining symptom strength by comparing a woman's ratings with a personal baseline may get around this problem. Using an individual baseline before assuming dysfunction within the menstrual cycle also accommodates the fact that women vary considerably in the degree to which they experience biological and behavioral symptoms defining menstrual disorders during the time when they are between menstrual periods. This would argue for a required deviation from ordinary experience as the woman approaches her period before assuming menstrual dysfunction. For example, if the person were quite tense as a regular thing, the report of tension during the premenstrual period would not point to menstrual dysfunction unless the rating was even higher.

Gruba and Rohrbaugh (1975) had suggested many years earlier than Logue and Moos (1986) that the MDQ score procedure should include a personal baseline of complaint, and they made specific recommendations on how this could be done. The symptom ratings for the intermenstrual period could be used as a reference point when considering level of distress during the premenstrual (week before flow) or menstrual (flow) periods. This would require that the woman report a considerable increment of distress associated with the approach or actuality of menstruation beyond her "normal" experience before symptom scores would be elevated to the point where subclinical PMS or dysmenorrhea would be suspected.

We availed ourselves of these suggestions by defining the subject's final premenstrual-distress score by a sum of her symptom ratings, as experienced during this 7-day span before menstrual flow, minus the sum of these ratings for the intermenstrual interval. The menstrual-distress score was determined in the same way by subtracting the sum of the intermenstrual symptom ratings from the menstrual sum score. These distress scores, corrected for individual level of complaint and experience, gave us a general sense of who was at-risk for serious menstrual dysfunction. Higher corrected menstrual-distress scores were adopted as a general indicator of symptomatic risk for dysmenorrhea, and higher corrected premenstrual-distress scores served as an indicator of symptomatic risk for PMS.

Menstrual Cycle Dysfunction and Stress: The Research Evidence

The research into early risk factors in PMS and dysmenorrhea, as far as it went, took advantage of the disclosures regarding stress and other specific risk variables provided by earlier investigations. Cognitive and social aspects of personality that showed promise in establishing risk for anorexia nervosa or coronary-prone Type A status were introduced into studies of menstrual dysfunction. The particular variables chosen for study also seemed relevant to the problems facing women who anticipate or experience problems in menstruation. These included self-preoccupation, psychological defenses, and sex-role commitment.

Self-preoccupation, stress, and menstrual cycle dysfunction. Self-preoccupation, the tendency to invest concern in oneself as opposed to others, was identified as an important risk factor in anorectic development. In fact, self-directed concern has been identified as the one cognitive attribute that might qualify as a "master trait" in the development of all stress-related disorders. Self-preoccupation not only seems to promote stress by itself but also seems capable of influencing the strength of other traits that govern the level of stress experienced by the at-risk individual.

The basis of self-preoccupation for the woman at anorectic risk can be traced most obviously to her fixation upon the size and contour of her body along with the effects of eating as they impact upon the body. A similar basis for self-preoccupation as part of the risk pattern in menstrual dysfunction suggests itself. Suffering associated with the menstrual cycle fixes the attention of the woman upon her own body and bodily functions. I will extend upon the basis for self-preoccupation as we cover the Type A in the chapters ahead; bodily concerns do not play a central role in this personality pattern.

Heilbrun and Frank (1989) considered self-preoccupation as a risk factor in menstrual dysfunction based on the reasoning that the more self-preoccupied woman would be more sensitive to aversive changes associated with menstruation because of her added vigilance. Hypervigilance would lead the woman to a heightened experience of distressing symptoms.

Stress also was considered as a possible collaborative factor in premenstrual or menstrual distress by Heilbrun and Frank. Previous researchers had pointed out that psychological stress may enhance distress experienced during the premenstrual phase (Clare, 1979; Damas-Mora, Davies, Taylor & Jenner, 1980; Morse & Dennerstein, 1988) or increase symptom severity during menstrual flow, at least in women suffering from spasmodic dysmenorrhea (Amos & Khanna, 1985). The effects of stress would be expected to combine with changes within the menstrual cycle; the reader may recall that there is a considerable overlap in symptoms between stress and menstrual change so that more profound distress would result. The increased sensitivity brought about by self-preoccupation would further magnify this blend of symptoms.

Stress and self-preoccupation would contribute to dysfunctional menstruation in different ways as may already be clear. Stress should add to the severity of changes and self-preoccupation should increase sensitivity and decrease tolerance. The combination of faulty menstrual functioning, self-preoccupation, and high stress would increase the risk of serious disorder within the menstrual cycle.

The methodology of this investigation holds no surprises. Premenstrual distress and menstrual distress were determined from the MDQ using the personal-baseline scoring procedure discussed previously. Self-preoccupation was measured by the self-schema laboratory procedure, and stress was gauged from the checklist of symptoms experienced on a daily basis. The sample included 55 college females.

The questions of whether self-preoccupation or life stress serve to enhance dysfunctional symptoms during the premenstrual or menstrual periods were considered in stages. Analysis of the evidence was guided by the fact that we were trying to improve understanding of risk for two disorders rather than one, not unlike our interest in distinguishing anorectic and bulimic risk treated earlier in the book. After determining the corrected PMS and corrected dysmenorrhea risk scores for each subject, the first analysis compared the degree of self-preoccupation and stress found in women who report three patterns of menstrual change: (1) those who rate premenstrual symptoms as more salient than menstrual symptoms, (2) those who indicate menstrual symptoms to be more distressing than premenstrual symptoms, and (3) those who report premenstrual and menstrual symptoms as essentially identical in strength. Assignment of subjects to these three pattern groups began by subtracting menstrual-distress scores from premenstrual-distress scores for all subjects. This distribution of difference scores for the 55 women was then separated into thirds. The upper third of the subjects had premenstrual-distress scores that exceeded menstrual-distress scores by 14.71 on the average. These women were identified as more at-risk for a PMS disorder. The average discrepancies for the subjects who had roughly equivalent premenstrual and menstrual symptom ratings was .37, and they represented a non-risk control group. Women in the lower third of the distribution presented menstrual-distress ratings that surpassed those obtained at the premenstrual stage by an average of 17.58. This group was considered at greater risk for dysmenorrhea. Looked at another way, the PMS risk group presented an average corrected premenstrual score of 35.29, and an average corrected menstrual score of 24.68 was obtained for the dysmenorrhea risk group. The control group of women obtained corrected premenstrual and menstrual symptom scores that averaged 12.79 and 13.16, respectively.

Table 6.1 discloses the average stress and self-preoccupation figures for the three symptom-pattern groups. The PMS risk group reported a general stress level well above that of the control and dysmenorrhea risk groups which, in turn, presented almost identical low stress scores. Statistics did not confirm significant variation in stress among the three independent groups, but if the PMS risk group is compared to the other look-alike groups combined, a significant difference appears ($p < .05$). Women reporting extraordinary changes during the week preceding menstruation also describe themselves as uniquely exposed to daily stress in their lives compared to the rest of the sample. The self-preoccupation variable provided a similar but more definitive picture as all three scores varied widely ($p < .001$). The PMS risk group was more self-preoccupied than the controls ($p < .001$) or the group at-risk for dysmenorrhea ($p < .01$). The latter two subsets of college women did not differ in self-preoccupation from each other. Self-preoccupation, then, was a prominent feature in college women whose dysfunctional symptoms were primarily confined to the premenstrual period. This opening analysis confirmed both stress and self-preoccupation as PMS risk factors but not as warning signs in dysmenorrhea.

Having considered self-preoccupation and stress independently as risk factors, we turned to examining their joint relationship in determining vulnerability to dysfunction within the menstrual cycle. One approach was to consider how stress level varied when the three symptom-pattern groups were broken down by self-preoccupation level. A median split on the sample score distribution was used to distinguish high and low self-preoccupation. Table 6.2 presents the average stress reported by the resulting six groups. The only reliable overall effect within the Table 6.2 data was an interaction ($p < .05$). Women at-risk for PMS who demonstrate high self-preoccupation stand alone in reported stress ($M = 54.15$). This level of stress was well above that reported by the few women with predominant premenstrual symptoms and low self-preoccupation ($M = 23.25$, $p < .01$). The enhancing effect of self-preoccupation upon stress failed to appear in the control and predominant menstrual-symptom groups. In fact, the opposite trend can be noted, although not to a significant degree.

The Table 6.2 data place the combined role of self-preoccupation and stress in sharper focus with regard to the risk ahead for more serious PMS problems. Prior analysis had confirmed the common presence of higher stress and greater self-preoccupation in college women with predominant premenstrual-distress scores. This analysis

Table 6.1.   Risk Factors in College Women with Greater
Premenstrual[a] or Menstrual[b] Distress

	Distress Group		
	Premenstrual > Menstrual (N = 17)	Premenstrual = Menstrual (N = 19)	Menstrual > Premenstrual (N = 19)
Added Risk Factor	M	M	M
General Stress	48.06	37.79	38.53
Self-preoccupation	56.82	15.47	26.74

Note. - Adapted from Heilbrun, A. B., & Frank, M. E. (1989). Self-preoccupation and general stress level as sensitizing factors in premenstrual and menstrual distress. Journal of Psychosomatic Research, 33, 571-577.
[a]Premenstrual = the week before menstrual flow.
[b]Menstrual = the period of menstrual flow.

Table 6.2   Level of General Stress Reported by College Women as a Function of Predominant Premenstrual or Menstrual Distress and Level of Self-preoccupation

| Level of Self-preoccupation | Distress Group | | | | | |
| | Premenstrual > Menstrual | | Premenstrual = Menstrual | | Menstrual > Premenstrual | |
	N	M	N	M	N	M
High	13	54.15	6	31.17	9	37.89
Low	4	23.25	13	40.85	10	39.10

Note. - Adapted from Heilbrun, A. B., & Frank, M. E. (1989). Self-preoccupation and general stress level as sensitizing factors in premenstrual and menstrual distress. Journal of Psychosomatic Research, 33, 571-577.

identified high self-preoccupation as a necessary condition for elevated stress but only in the PMS risk group. The present analysis also made it clear that most of the women at-risk for PMS (76%) were self-preoccupied.

A second approach to evaluating the relationship between self-preoccupation, stress, and primary menstrual or premenstrual dysfunction was considered. It involved examination of the combined effects of the two specific risk factors, self-preoccupation and stress, upon symptomatic changes reported for these discrete periods within the menstrual cycle. As the reader can see, this represents an analysis of the same three risk variables turned around as dependent and independent variables. We did not want to ignore any possibility given the results reported to this point. We had not initiated the investigation of risk for menstrual-cycle dysfunction with the expectation that such clearcut findings would appear for PMS risk and nothing would be found for the risk of dysmenorrhea.

Sample medians on the self-preoccupation and stress distributions were used as cutting points to assign subjects to risk groups. Perhaps needless to say, the women high on self-preoccupation and high on stress represented those at highest risk for dysfunction within the menstrual cycle. Table 6.3 offers the corrected premenstrual-symptom scores and menstrual-symptom scores for the four risk groups.

There was no overall effect revealed by statistical analysis of the premenstrual-symptom scores across risk groups, although the premenstrual distress for women displaying both high self-preoccupation and high stress ($M = 30.43$) was far higher than that reported by any other group of women. This is often the fate of a deeply-embedded effect when overall effects are examined. It was possible to show that this higher level of premenstrual distress for the group at highest risk was significantly above that of the remaining three risk groups combined ($M = 13.44$, $p < .05$).

The overall analysis of menstrual distress failed to disclose any effect of self-preoccupation and stress. In addition, parallel extreme-group analysis involving comparison of menstrual-symptom scores of women with both risk factors operative ($M = 24.07$) did not reveal a reliable difference from these scores reported by the remainder of the sample ($M = 17.83$). Examination of Table 6.3 does offer a hint of an effect within the menstrual-symptom scores if only the extreme risk groups are considered. The college women with low self-preoccupation and low stress, both risk factors absent, reported the least menstrual dis-

Table 6.3. Levels of Premenstrual Distress and Menstrual Distress in College Women as a Function of Self-preoccupation and Stress

| | Level of Self-Preoccupation | | | |
| | High | | Low | |
Type of Distress	High Stress (N = 14) M	Low Stress (N = 15) M	High Stress (N = 14) M	Low Stress (N = 12) M
Premenstrual	30.43	23.00	9.50	11.33
Menstrual	24.07	23.00	18.07	11.08

Note. - Adapted from Heilbrun, A. B., & Frank, M. E. (1989). Self-preoccupation and general stress level as sensitizing factors in premenstrual and menstrual distress. Journal of Psychosomatic Research, 33, 571-577.

tress ($\underline{M}$ = 11.08). When this low symptom score was compared with the $\underline{M}$ = 24.07 figure of the highest risk group, the difference was significant ($\underline{p}$ < .05). Given this much statistical license, it was possible to show that the combination of self-preoccupation and stress was associated with greater menstrual distress. Nevertheless, it remains clear that the impact of these specific risk variables was less robust in our data when changes during menstrual flow were examined than was true when the premenstrual period was considered.

Recapitulating these results, higher self-preoccupation emerged as a clearcut risk factor for women whose problems within the menstrual cycle are concentrated in the premenstrual period. Stress effects were more difficult to demonstrate, although women with dominant premenstrual distress did report higher stress than all other groups combined. The role of stress was more clearly defined when it was considered in combination with self-preoccupation. Women at-risk for PMS who were highly self-preoccupied also maintained a heavy burden of stress unmatched by any other segment of women in the sample. The coalescence of risk factors that attracted so much attention in our studies of anorectic vulnerability -- self-preoccupation and stress -- was evident only in subjects who had begun to experience distress in the week prior to menstrual flow. A final analysis in which we turned our variables around did disclose one new effect, although it was rather weak. Those women who demonstrated both specific risk variables did report more severe symptoms during menstruation than others who did not demonstrate either high self-preoccupation or elevated stress.

Psychological defenses and menstrual cycle dysfunction.   Each of our programs of research into stress-related disorder has included an investigation of psychological defenses. The research question in each case has been whether particular cognitive strategies of self-protection against threatening information are more maladaptive than others, thereby increasing the woman's vulnerability to a given disorder. The verdict in the study bearing upon anorectic risk was that the most evasive defense, repression, was a preferred mode of defense in women with a high anorectic profile (Heilbrun & Harris, 1986). Projection was generally avoided as a defense mechanism by these same women and came to be viewed as a contraindication of risk.

Repressive tendencies to put disturbing thoughts out of mind and to avoid remembering them was viewed as promoting poorer problem resolution. The failure to resolve problems of attainment in the repressive but ambitious college female makes it likely that stress will continue. The stress-maintenance role of repression qualified it as an anorectic risk factor in my conceptual framework, since the attempt to cope with the stress of being a nonachiever in her own eyes leads the at-risk female toward a substitute goal of bodily thinness and compensatory dieting.

To gauge the contribution of defenses to the risk of menstrual or premenstrual disorder requires that we go one step beyond the issue of evasiveness and consider at greater length why being evasive can be maladjustive to begin with. The more that the defense distances the person from a distressing event or situation, the less likely that direct efforts to resolve the source of stress will be taken. The key assumption here is that the stressor can be modified by taking direct action. However, if little or nothing can be done to modify a stressor by direct action, at least in the view of the person under stress, coping by psychological defenses may take on added importance and the adaptive priorities among the strategies of defense may shift.

Menstruation seemed to represent a potentially stressful event in the lives of many women that would be regularly occurring and difficult to modify by direct means if it proved a source of problems. Given the more immutable quality of menstruation and whatever level of discomfort that is associated with it, the question of which defenses play a significant role in stress management, for better or for worse, became a matter of interest. The Heilbrun and Renert (1988) study offered a look at the defenses of 81 college women who also reported upon their premenstrual and menstrual symptoms.

The study of relationships between defenses and menstrual and premenstrual distress involved the MDQ measure of symptoms (using the correction by intermenstrual score as described previously) along with the standard laboratory procedures for estimating the strength of four defenses -- repression, projection, rationalization, and denial. Defense awareness scores also were introduced into the Heilbrun and Renert study. We had failed to take this precaution in the investigation of defenses and anorectic risk (Heilbrun & Harris, 1986), although the relationships came through even without the added power of an awareness measure. Repression without awareness proved to be a more stress-provoking pattern in several other studies just as rationalization without awareness turned out to be associated with the least stress in college students.

Awareness of any given defense was determined by the correspondence between the subject's actual performance on the laboratory task measuring that defense and her rating of everyday use made of that particular strategy of deflecting distressing information. If she were high (above the sample median) on the well-disguised laboratory measure for a defense and yet stated that she made little use of that defense (below the sample median), she was considered "unaware." The correspondence between defensive performance and rated usage also defined awareness or unawareness for other combinations: high actual use-high rated use, "aware"; low actual use-high rated use, "unaware"; low actual use-low rated use, "aware."

College women high and low on each of the four defenses (repression, projection, rationalization, denial) relative to the sample median were further subdivided by mid-point for level of awareness. The defense x awareness groupings were analyzed separately for both corrected menstrual-distress and premenstrual-distress scores. This analysis disclosed significant results for rationalization on both the menstrual-distress and premenstrual-distress scores; no hint of differences was found for the other defenses. Accordingly, Table 6.4 includes only the rationalization findings. One significant effect ($\underline{p} < .05$) indicated that subjects high in rationalization and unaware of it were less inclined ($\underline{p} < .05$) to experience menstrual distress ($\underline{M} = 21.71$) than rationalizers who indicated awareness of this defensive strategy ($\underline{M} = 37.67$).

The other women in the sample, who failed to display a rationalizing style of defense, did not vary in reported menstrual problems whether they were cognizant of their restricted use of rationalization or not.

The Table 6.4 data concerned with premenstrual distress offered the same conclusion when subjected to analysis. Distress within the week preceding menstrual flow varied with level of rationalizing defense and awareness. Rationalizers who were unaware of using this defense revealed less in the way of premenstrual symptoms ($\underline{M} = 12.10$) than women who used rationalization but were more aware of what they were doing ($\underline{M} = 29.14$, $\underline{p} < .05$). Awareness level among low rationalizers had no effect upon reported premenstrual symptoms.

Both sets of results identify unconscious rationalization as a risk factor for disorders of the menstrual cycle, but it was the failure to take advantage of this pattern of defense that served as a marker of vulnerability. No other defense, considered by level of awareness, showed a relationship to menstrual and premenstrual distress and promise as an indicator of risk. The implications of these findings will be considered

Table 6.4   Menstrual and Premenstrual Distress for College Women as a Function of a Rationalizing Defense and Level of Awareness

Rationalizing Defense and Awareness Pattern	Menstrual Distress	Premenstrual Distress
	$\underline{M}$	$\underline{M}$
High Rationalization		
Aware ($\underline{N}$ = 21)	37.67	29.14
Unaware ($\underline{N}$ = 20)	21.71	12.10
Low Rationalization		
Aware ($\underline{N}$ = 19)	34.64	25.00
Unaware ($\underline{N}$ = 21)	28.00	23.48

Note. - Adapted from Heilbrun, A. B., & Renert, D. (1988). Psychological defenses and menstrual distress. British Journal of Medical Psychology, 61, 219-230.

after further evidence from the Heilbrun and Renert study is presented.

I pointed out earlier in the book that the at-risk research strategy was geared to discovering risk factors and their patterns among normals that would have a bearing on who might later demonstrate one or another stress-related disorder. The eventual confirmation of these risk factors by studying actual clinical cases was considered to be of future importance, especially if longitudinal research procedures were possible. The Heilbrun and Renert study of defenses and menstrual risk proved to be the only exception to this dictum in the programs of research into stress and disorder. We collected a small sample of women from the community to see whether unconscious rationalization (or its absence) was a factor in women suffering from PMS. These subjects were obtained through the cooperation of an Atlanta PMS support group and included women who had received a PMS diagnosis and others whom they recruited and who reported normal menstrual cycles. Although the number of volunteers we were able to recruit fell below minimum standards for population sampling, the evidence on rationalization was powerful enough to compel attention anyway.

The 12 PMS and 7 control women were reasonably well matched on average age (35-37 years), average education (three years of college), current marriage (57%-69%), and current employment (69%-100%). These community subjects completed the MDQ, defensive tasks, and the ratings of everyday use of the defenses. The average corrected premenstrual-distress score for the PMS subjects was 89.92 compared to a mean of 13.57 for the controls; the difference was highly reliable ($p < .001$) and verified their group assignments. Corrected menstrual distress scored from the MDQ showed an average of 46.58 for PMS females compared to a mean of 14.71 for controls. Despite the seeming discrepancy in means, statistical test revealed no difference between PMS and control groups for symptom severity during menstrual flow.

Tables 6.3 and 6.4, presented earlier, include no average symptom scores for college women at-risk for PMS that are near the figures provided by the PMS women from the community. This observation confirms what we already assumed to be true. Our college subjects, even those thought to be most seriously at-risk for future clinical disorders of menstruation, do not match the intensity of symptoms found in women who actually suffer from disorder. The marked discrepancy in corrected premenstrual-distress scores on the MDQ between the PMS group and at-risk college females supports the assumption of a transitional stage where discomforting symptoms signal risk but not full-blown disorder.

In order to consider whether the rationalization findings could be replicated with such small samples, the 12 PMS women were divided into only two subgroups -- those who could be defined as unconscious rationalizers ($\underline{N}$ = 5) and those who could not ($\underline{N}$ = 7). These assignments were based upon whether or not the woman fell above the mid-point on the rationalization score for the PMS group while falling below the mid-point on reported usage of that defense (i.e., unconscious rationalization). Table 6.5 includes the corrected symptom scores for the two PMS subgroups and for controls without respect to defensive style. A significant decrement in premenstrual distress ($\underline{p}$ < .05) was confirmed when the PMS women utilizing unconscious rationalization ($\underline{M}$ = 67.00) were compared to the rest of the PMS group ($\underline{M}$ = 106.29). Even within a group of women identified as suffering from PMS, the distress during the premenstrual period was demonstrably less if rationalization was a defensive strategy of choice and the woman lacked cognizance of its use.

The same statistical procedure applied to the menstrual-symptom means in Table 6.5 brought the same result. Unconscious rationalizers reported less distress during menses ($\underline{M}$ = 16.00) than other PMS women ($\underline{M}$ = 68.43, $\underline{p}$ < .05). In fact, rationalizing PMS women, unaware of this defensive style, looked normal in their level of distress during the period of menstruation. Inspection revealed no hint of association between any other defense/awareness pattern and premenstrual or menstrual symptoms. However, no pattern appeared in sufficient number to make statistical analysis worthwhile.

A final comment is in order regarding the study of community women actually suffering a PMS disorder. I already have conceded that the number of subjects included in the sample is small, something which automatically triggers concern about reliability of the results. Would the same results be found if a new sample were collected? This does not seem to be cause for concern in this case. For one thing, the results were predictable based upon the study of risk in college students and not an out-of-the-blue effect that might be random. For another, the opposite case seems more justified. The fact that predicted results could be demonstrated in such a small sample even with PMS symptom scores that were highly variable testifies to the power of the relationship between unconscious rationalization and reduced symptoms for PMS women.

Stress was not ignored as a risk factor in the Heilbrun and Renert

Table 6.5   Premenstrual and Menstrual Distress Scores for PMS Women With and Without Unconscious Rationalization Pattern of Defense and for Controls Reporting Normal Menstrual Cycles

Menstrual Phase	PMS Women		Control Women
	With Defense Pattern ($\underline{N}$ = 5)	Without Defense Pattern ($\underline{N}$ = 7)	Without Respect to Defense Pattern ($\underline{N}$ = 7)
	$\underline{M}$	$\underline{M}$	$\underline{M}$
Premenstrual	67.00	106.29	13.57
Menstrual	16.00	68.43	14.71

Note. - Adapted from Heilbrun, A. B., & Renert, D. (1988). Psychological defenses and menstrual distress. British Journal of Medical Psychology, 61, 219-230.

study of menstrual dysfunction in college women. I have postponed discussion of the stress-symptom scores until now in order to more firmly establish the role of unconscious rationalization in counteracting menstrual problems. Previous research with college students has shown rationalization to be a constructive mode of defense in terms of adjustment (Heilbrun, 1982); better adjustment should pay off in terms of reduced stress. Other studies in a college student population have directly confirmed the lower stress levels that accompany rationalization without awareness as well as the stress-promoting qualities of unconscious repression (Heilbrun, 1984; Heilbrun & Pepe, 1985). It was expected that the risk of premenstrual or menstrual disorder associated with style of defense, as evident from level of stress, would fall in line with the risk findings reported in the college and clinical samples. Unconscious rationalizers should show less stress to be consistent with the results reported to this point.

The analysis of stress reported by Heilbrun and Renert in their 1988 paper was surprisingly noncommittal as far as our understanding of risk was concerned. College women in the sample who qualified as unconscious rationalizers reported about the same level of stress as the rest of the subjects combined. The reduced stress load associated with unconscious rationalization in earlier studies was not in evidence. This apparent inconsistency was cleared up by a form of extreme-group comparison when only the subjects who were most certain about their everyday use of rationalization were included. Women who strenuously denied ever using rationalization (ratings of 0-1) were considered along with those who reported heavy usage (ratings of 5-6). The retention of only those who were most certain of how much they used rationalization resulted in 12 unconscious rationalizers and 37 women who did not demonstrate this defensive pattern. The stress level of women who employed rationalization without awareness ($\underline{M}$ = 31.67) fell well below that of the comparison group ($\underline{M}$ = 47.16). This difference ($\underline{p}$ < .05) was in line with prior evidence. Obviously, our measurement of the perceived use of rationalization lacked precision in this study once we got away from subjects who were more certain of themselves.

Recapitulating the Heilbrun and Renert findings to this point, the absence of unconscious rationalization has been confirmed as a risk factor in menstrual cycle dysfunction within two sets of women -- those in college and others living in the community who suffer from a PMS disorder. Low stress has been identified as a correlate of this critical defensive pattern using extreme-group analysis within the college sample. We next considered whether these specific risk factors coalesce in their effects with both unconscious rationalization and low stress serving to reduce the risk of menstrual disorder. Coalescence would lead us to expect lower menstrual and premenstrual distress if the subjects present both counterrisk factors than when rationalization without awareness or low stress appear singly or are both absent.

This analysis of factor patterning seemed especially important, because it was uncertain how the rationalizing defense and low stress would function to counteract menstrual and premenstrual distress by my theoretical assumptions. On the one hand, it could be reasoned that the defense pattern simply serves as the basis for less stress which, in turn, was the sole factor responsible for more comfortable menstrual-cycle functioning. Alternatively, somewhat independent contributions of rationalization without awareness and lower stress to less discomforting cyclical functioning might be anticipated if the defense pattern influenced cyclic discomfort in two ways. For example, the woman might rationalize her distress during the menstrual cycle as the price she had to pay for conceiving children. Unaware that she is distorting information, this rationalization of distress should improve the woman's tolerance of the symptoms and decrease her sensitivity. The defense, in other words, could make a contribution directly by increasing tolerance thresholds. Lower stress, routinely accompanying this defensive pattern, could make its independent contribution as a counterrisk factor by limiting the infusion of disagreeable stress components into the distress generated by the menstrual cycle itself. The defense pattern in this example would not only increase tolerance of menstrual distress directly but indirectly reduce the amount of distress to be tolerated.

This analysis of counterrisk factors in premenstrual and menstrual distress proceeded by taking sample characteristics into consideration. I knew that we had to use rating extremes in the previous examination of stress in order to reveal expected correlates of rationalization without awareness. It was clear from those data that an extreme of unconscious rationalization might be required to test for combined effects with stress. My choice was to measure unconscious rationalization as a single score and use this index to separate the sample of women into a middle group and two extremes -- those who were high on this defense pattern, those very low, and an intermediate group. Both the rationalization score and the rating score concerning everyday use of this defense were converted to the same kind of standard score distribution in such a way that higher rationalization scores and lower ratings of usage received higher transformed scores. These transformed scores were introduced into a multiplicative index; a woman with a higher rationalization score from the laboratory and lower awareness that she used this defense would earn an especially high index score. These index scores were split into three levels of equal size. Stress scores, in turn, were divided into high/low by separation at their sample midpoint.

Table 6.6 presents the corrected premenstrual-distress and menstrual-distress scores for the six unconscious rationalization x stress groupings. The most deviant results provided by this table involved the group with both counterrisk factors present. Females whose high use of unconscious rationalization brought about the low stress that we had come to expect also reported very little menstrual distress (M = 15.81). This level of distress during menses was less than all other groups, and far less than high unconscious rationalizers with high stress (M = 41.18, p < .01). At the remaining two levels of this defense pattern, level of stress was unrelated to menstrual distress. Avoidance of symptoms during menstruation required the presence of both counterrisk factors.

Premenstrual-distress results were very similar to those already considered for menstrual distress except they were a bit less robust. A difference was found between the low level of premenstrual discomfort found for women demonstrating high unconscious rationalization and low stress (M = 12.88) and that reported by women showing the same defense style but high stress (M = 26.09, p < .05). Nothing significant was forthcoming when stress levels were compared for women less given to using rationalization without awareness. Being less beset by stress was of no advantage in curtailing premenstrual and menstrual symptoms unless it accompanied the other counterrisk factor, unconscious rationalization.

The conclusion from this analysis of combined effects seems straightforward. Rationalization, given that the woman is relatively unaware that it is being employed as a strategy of defense, works in combination with lower stress levels to diminish the severity of problems encountered in the menstrual cycle. This defense pattern is capable of decreasing sensitivity to symptoms directly by offering a basis for greater tolerance. It also has an indirect influence on symptoms, since it helps to keep symptom-enhancing stress in check better than other defenses. If my reasoning is correct, this dual role would

Table 6.6.   Combined Effects of Unconscious Rationalization and Stress in Premenstrual and Menstrual Distress

	Unconscious Rationalization Level					
	High		Intermediate		Low	
	High Stress (N = 12)	Low Stress (N = 16)	High Stress (N = 15)	Low Stress (N = 11)	High Stress (N = 13)	Low Stress (N = 14)
Distress Variable	M	M	M	M	M	M
Premenstrual	26.09	12.88	21.12	25.82	20.50	22.86
Menstrual	41.18	15.81	30.75	36.27	29.38	31.43

Note. - Adapted from Heilbrun, A. B., & Renert, D. (1988). Psychological defenses and menstrual distress. British Journal of Medical Psychology, 61, 219-230.

qualify unconscious rationalization as especially important in counteracting cyclic distress.

Sex-role commitment and menstrual cycle dysfunction. A clear link existed between female sex-role status and menstrual functioning according to earlier psychoanalytic papers (Abraham, 1948; Balint, 1937; Benedek, 1959; Deutsch, 1944; Kestenberg, 1961; Menninger, 1939). The menstrual cycle, as the quintessential defining feature of the female role through its unique contribution to conception and reproduction, was thought to confirm the woman's femininity. According to these earlier scholars, rejection of femininity would lead the woman to resent menstrual changes; intolerance of menstruation would increase her chances of dysfunction within the reproductive system.

The research literature has not been kind to the proposed relationship between female alienation from the traditional feminine sex-role and menstrual or premenstrual dysfunction, although it is difficult to establish whether the problem rests with the idea or the fragmented research. The literature relating sex-role preferences of the woman to degree of cyclic dysfunction is next to chaotic in that investigators, working independently with varying methodologies, have produced substantial evidence that confirms seemingly opposite conclusions. Studies have emphasized two aspects of the woman's role, sex-role behavior and sex-role attitudes, and this division of interest may have added to the confusion.

Investigations concerned with sex-role behavior have directed their attention to the fit between the woman's actual manifest behavior and culturally-prescribed expectations for the female role (femininity) or the male role (masculinity). Some of these studies have disclosed that it is the feminine woman who is vulnerable to menstrual distress (Chernovetz, Jones & Hansson, 1979; Gough, 1975; Meltzer, 1974; Paige, 1973; Peshkin, 1968). However, just as commonly negative results have cast doubt upon a relationship between femininity and menstrual problems (Greenberg & Fisher, 1984; Gruba & Rohrbaugh, 1975; Haft, 1973; Shader & Ohly, 1970; Slade & Jenner, 1980). Masculinity also has been related to menstrual dysfunction (Good & Smith, 1980; Greenberg & Fisher, 1984; Woods & Launius, 1979), but disconfirming evidence has been found here as well (Chernovetz et al., 1979; Herzberg, 1970).

Numerous studies dealing with sex-role attitudes present the same inconsistency. Contemporary role attitudes generally favor abolishing differences in the male and female roles -- career opportunities should be equated, home and child-care responsibilities more evenly shared, etc. Evidence has shown that contemporary women are more vulnerable to menstrual distress (Berry & McGuire, 1972; Paulson, 1956; Shainess, 1961; Spero, 1968). The traditional view of the woman's role sets it apart from the male role and emphasizes marital and family responsibilities. Women with traditional role attitudes have been reported as more prone to menstrual dysfunction just as often as their contemporary counterparts (Brattesceni & Silverthorne, 1978; Olds & Shaver, 1980; Schneider & Schneider-Duker, 1974; Woods, 1985). As might be evident, sex-role commitment, whether measured by attitude or manifest behavior, holds an elusive relationship with problems of menstruation.

Heilbrun, Friedberg, Wydra, and Worobow (1990) published a conceptual and methodological inquiry into the abundant inconsistencies within the literature relating the woman's role to menstrual disorder. Their study was not focused directly upon the identification of risk factors that occupies my interest in this book. Accordingly, I will abstract the substantive evidence from this study without dwelling upon the implications regarding research methodology emphasized in the original paper. However, before I direct your attention to the sex-role risk factors in menstrual and premenstrual disorder, it will be necessary to consider at least one of the methodological issues that was ignored in prior investigations, at least to my knowledge. This exception must be made, because the resolution of the issue determined how the risk data will be presented.

Some prior research had considered whether problems during the menstrual cycle were related to traditional feminine role behavior in the woman or to a more masculine commitment. Alternatively, other investigators had examined the relationships between menstrual-cycle dysfunction and traditional or contemporary sex-role attitudes. Correspondence or lack of correspondence between behavior and attitudes had not attracted the attention of researchers in their quest for correlates of dysfunction. Perhaps it was assumed that women who behave in a more traditional feminine way would automatically hold traditional sex-role attitudes or that more masculine women must necessarily share contemporary attitudes. The seemingly logical assumption of a syncronous relationship between role behavior and role attitudes is not supported by the evidence, as shall be seen.

The Heilbrun, Friedberg, Wydra, and Worobow paper reported two studies in which various combinations of sex-role behavior (feminine/masculine) and attitudes toward the woman's role (traditional/contemporary) were related to premenstrual and menstrual symptoms. In the original sample of 49 college females, sex-role categories of predominantly masculine (masculine score > feminine score) and predominantly feminine (feminine score > masculine score) were created from the independent scales of masculinity and femininity provided by the Bem Sex Role Inventory (Bem 1981b). The scores on the Attitude Toward Women scale (Spence, Helmreich, & Stapp, 1973; 1975), divided at their median, were used to identify women with more contemporary or more traditional attitudes. Four groups were constituted from these divisions -- contemporary-masculine, contemporary-feminine, traditional-masculine, and traditional-feminine. The replication sample of 96 college women used identical assignment procedures for the sex-role attitude/behavior groupings. The fact that behaviors and attitudes are often inconsistent is made apparent by the substantial number of women who reported predominantly feminine behavior but more contemporary attitudes or predominantly masculine behavior and more traditional attitudes (see Table 6.7).

The corrected MDQ menstrual-symptom and premenstrual-symptom scores for the four role groups within the original and replication samples are reported in Table 6.7. Statistical findings for the original and replication analyses were very similar. The initial analysis revealed an interaction between predominant sex-role behavior and role attitudes for the menstrual-distress score ($p < .01$) and for the premenstrual-distress scores ($p < .05$). The replication sample provided an interaction for the menstrual-distress variable ($p < .001$) and a nearly-significant interaction ($p < .10$) for premenstrual symptoms.

The interpretation of statistical results for Table 6.7 data would be the same for both samples of college women. Female subjects who are consistent in their role attitudes and sex-role behavior report the highest level of menstrual and premenstrual distress. Thus, women who preferred contemporary role values and who described their behavior as predominantly masculine, along with women who adhered to more traditional role values and who reported a predominantly feminine identity, experienced more severe symptoms before and during menstruation. Subjects who went through less premenstrual and menstrual distress presented an inconsistency in their commitment to the woman's role -- contemporary attitudes accompanied by more feminine behavior or traditional attitudes with more masculine behavior. In the original paper these replicated interaction effects were used to

Table 6.7.   Role Correlates of Menstrual and Premenstrual Distress in Two Samples of College Women

Sample and Type of Distress	Contemporary Attitudes		Traditional Attitudes	
	More Masculine Than Feminine Behavior M	More Feminine Than Masculine Behavior M	More Masculine Than Feminine Behavior M	More Feminine Than Masculine Behavior M
Original Sample	(N = 15)	(N = 10)	(N = 8)	(N = 16)
Menstrual	33.33	14.50	18.12	36.44
Premenstrual	25.53	7.20	15.25	29.94
Replication Sample	(N = 16)	(N = 22)	(N = 25)	(N = 33)
Menstrual	29.06	18.91	19.68	28.76
Premenstrual	26.25	18.42	14.96	22.88

Note. - Adapted from Heilbrun, A. B., Friedberg, L., Wydra, D., & Worobow, A. L. (1990). The female role and menstrual distress. Psychology of Women Quarterly, 14, 403-417.

mount an obvious methodological warning for this kind of research into menstrual dysfunction. Consider both role variables or risk cultivating unreliable results.

The role findings considered in the context of discovering premenstrual and menstrual risk factors are readily interpreted up to a point. The college woman who is more fully committed to the values and behaviors of the traditional feminine role or to the values and behaviors of masculinity is at greater risk of premenstrual or menstrual disorder. This represents a straightforward reading of the replicated statistical interactions and falls short of any dynamic explanation of why "pure" role types should share a common vulnerability to distress within the menstrual cycle. While extensive speculation does not seem warranted for what could prove to be a very complicated psychobiological phenomenon, some effort at explanation may bolster confidence in the role parameters of risk that were disclosed.

Let me begin by admitting that I did not expect the replicated results that were obtained. Inconsistency between sex-role attitudes and behavior was viewed as a more likely contributor to cyclic dysfunction. As a clinical psychologist, I was prepared to find conflict between role components and diminished role commitment to be at the roots of menstrual dysfunction, since my experience had taught me that incompatible or inconsistent behaviors are likely to generate stress. Stress, in turn, should adversely affect menstrual functioning by combining with the cycle-based symptoms. With the wisdom of hindsight and the fortunate inclusion of a role-conflict rating scale in the original study that was not considered in the methodological paper, I believe I can make the risk evidence more understandable.

The finding that more masculine college women with synchronous contemporary role values report higher levels of premenstrual and menstrual distress actually represents a belated validation of the psychoanalytic view concerning disorders of the menstrual cycle. This theory proposed that rejection of femininity could reduce the woman's tolerance for menstrual changes, since these changes symbolized her biological preparation for conception and reproduction that was at the heart of traditional female expectations. The intolerance of cyclical changes would make dysfunction more likely. In our study, the college women who could be said to have "rejected" femininity in the most complete sense are those who report masculine behavior and express contemporary values. These women were among those who were experiencing problems in the menstrual cycle. To use the terminology of our risk studies, the masculine/contemporary women would be sensitized to menstrual changes, since this biological system holds little priority; sensitivity to these changes magnifies their intensity, lowers the threshold of tolerance, and magnifies the subjective experience of discomfort.

Given rejection of femininity as key to problems in the menstrual cycle, how are we to explain the identical finding of cyclic distress in the most feminine of our subjects who meet traditional expectations by both behavior and attitude? Role conflict as a source of stress that augments the psychological and biological turmoil of menstrual changes offers one explanation. Role conflict, as used here, describes a state in which a woman feels she cannot achieve the desired goals associated with the traditional and contemporary roles for women, because attaining one tends to preclude attaining the other. Role conflict, should it exist, could arise under two distinct conditions. A woman with contemporary attitudes, determined to have a successful professional career, will feel that as a consequence she will not be able to marry or, at least, will not have a marriage that meets her expectations. Alternatively, a woman with traditional values, who is interested primarily in getting married and having a family, will feel that she cannot pursue a successful career. Role conflict, then, amounts to the feeling that optimal achievements of a career and marriage/family are to some degree incompatible and that one or the other goal must be relinquished or compromised. Since both career and marriage hold importance to most young-adult women in college, this sense of conflicted options for the future could be a fairly common source of stress.

Scores on a 9-point rating scale (Diller, 1986) of role conflict were analyzed within the initial 49-subject sample for the two higher-risk groups (masculine/contemporary and feminine/traditional) considered independently. The remaining subjects, who reported relatively little premenstrual or menstrual distress, were combined and served as controls. Role conflict results identified the feminine/traditional women as the most deeply concerned about the incompatibility between career and marriage ($\underline{M} = 6.12$, $\underline{N} = 16$). At the other extreme, masculine/contemporary females expressed the least concern about this future problem ($\underline{M} = 2.80$, $\underline{N} = 15$). Control women's ratings of role conflict fell in-between ($\underline{M} = 5.06$, $\underline{N} = 18$). These mean values varied significantly ($\underline{p} < .001$).

It is instructive to go beyond the fact that these role-conflict values differ statistically to take a look at the literal meanings of the scale rating points that are indicated by the average group scores. The low value for the masculine/traditional women portrays the conflict between career and marriage as falling short of qualifying as even "slightly important." College women who present a mix of masculine behavior with traditional values or feminine behavior with contemporary values chose "moderately important" to describe the personal relevance of role conflict on average. Traditional/feminine females emphasized the importance of role conflict by rating it midway between "moderately important" and "very important." It is clear that college women who fully conform to traditional role expectations are deeply concerned about a perceived conflict in options for a career as well as marriage and children.

These results offer an alternative explanation of premenstrual/ menstrual distress that would be suitable for the college woman who is traditional in behavior and attitude. The extent of their role conflict would be enough to generate stress as they approach the point in life, 18 years of age or slightly older, when this issue is a relevant concern. This is not to say that other critical sources of stress for the traditional college woman do not exist. It was not that many pages back that stress-related factors contributing to anorectic risk included a feminine sex-role preference and sensitivity to traditional role assignments. The feminine role in that case was considered to be a current barrier to effective competition for either career or social goals. More purely feminine college women have stress-provoking problems relating to the present as well as the future.

In these efforts to explain the duality of risk factors for menstrual and premenstrual disorders within the sex-role evidence, I have fallen back on the complementary principles of sensitization and augmentation again. In the case of the more purely masculine college women, cyclic changes are less readily tolerated, since the child-bearing functions of the cycle are of little immediate significance. With less tolerance comes sensitivity and an enhancement of menstrual and premenstrual discomfort. Reactive stress, of course, would be expected as the discomfort itself becomes a source of concern.

Women of more purely feminine commitment would not likely share the intolerance of the extremely masculine woman. Rather, they are vulnerable to the perceived conflict between career and marriage and to problems of competing for either goal. With conflict and limited competitiveness comes added stress for these feminine and traditional college women, and it is the stress burden that intrudes itself into the discomfort already attending cyclic changes.

Self-preoccupation and multiple risk for disorder. The possibility that a factor might mediate risk of more than one stress-related disorder for the same woman was considered by including the EDI in the test battery of the Heilbrun and Frank (1989) study. Even though the symptoms of anorexia nervosa had no clear bearing on the relationships between self-preoccupation, stress, and premenstrual/menstrual distress, there were reasons to believe that the EDI might prove informative as part of a follow-up analysis.

For one thing, the issue of multiple risk for anorectic and menstrual disorders deserved consideration in itself. The Heilbrun and Frank study gave us the opportunity to examine this point. The second basis for our interest in multiple risk was inherent in the self-preoccupation construct. Both the woman at anorectic risk and the woman experiencing premenstrual or menstrual problems had ample reason for self-preoccupation based upon body concerns. In the former case, the woman would be expected to dwell upon body form and in the latter case upon body function that feeds into and is enhanced by self-preoccupation. Sensitivity to her own body could enhance the risk of both types of disorder.

Heilbrun and Frank divided the scores on the self-schema task and the EDI for the 55 college women by their respective mid-points. This allowed them to separated their sample into high AP (at-risk) and control groups followed by high and low self-preoccupation. The four subgroups defined by these categorizations were then compared on the two corrected distress scores from the MDQ. These menstrual-distress and premenstrual-distress means are found in Table 6.8.

Examination of Table 6.8 data reveals that women at highest anorectic risk, high AP women who are self-preoccupied, were distinct from the remaining groups on both symptom scores. The remaining three AP/self-preoccupation combinations looked much alike. The self-preoccupied and high AP females reported greater menstrual distress (M = 27.00) than the remaining groups (Ms = 13.31-18.77) and surpassed their combined mean with statistical reliability (M = 15.16, p < .05). In the same vein, self-preoccupied females with elevated anorectic profiles described their premenstrual symptoms as more severe (M = 29.75) than did the remainder of the subjects (Ms = 10.15-14.10) and exceeded their combined average (M = 13.46, p < .05). These analyses suggest that college women who display the early symptoms that place them at-risk for anorexia are also generally at-risk for

Table 6.8. Menstrual and Premenstrual Distress Reported by Self-preoccupied College Women at Anorectic Risk and Their Controls

	Women at Anorectic Risk		Controls	
	High Self-preoccupation ($\underline{N}$ = 16)	Low Self-preoccupation ($\underline{N}$ = 13)	High Self-preoccupation ($\underline{N}$ = 10)	Low Self-preoccupation ($\underline{N}$ = 16)
Correlates	$\underline{M}$	$\underline{M}$	$\underline{M}$	$\underline{M}$
Menstrual Distress	27.00	18.77	16.60	13.31
Premenstrual Distress	29.75	10.15	14.10	13.50

Note. - From Heilbrun, A. B. & Frank, M. E. (1989). Self-preoccupation and general stress level as sensitizing factors in premenstrual and menstrual distress. Journal of Psychosomatic Research, 33, 571-577.

serious menstrual and premenstrual symptoms. This is true only if they are highly self-preoccupied, however. At some period prior to actual disorder, there does seem to be a common sensitivity to body form (thinness) and body function (menstrual changes) that puts the female in jeopardy of an anorectic disorder or a disorder of the menstrual cycle.

This convergence of risk factors seems to be at odds with the diagnostic specifications provided by DSM-III-R for anorexia nervosa. The findings just reported regarding multiple risk would lead us to expect self-preoccupied women who are predisposed toward anorexia to experience distressing levels of premenstrual and menstrual symptoms. The diagnostic manual calls for changes in menstruation as part of the anorectic symptom picture, but these involve cessation of menstrual flow rather than active symptomatology preceding or accompanying actual menstrual flow. The drastic food reduction accompanying restraint during the risk period and the semi-starvation of anorexia nervosa brings about a cessation of menstrual flow. If our multiple-risk findings are correct, the self-preoccupied woman suffering from anorexia nervosa will have yet another incentive for maintaining her food restriction. She may have found a way of avoiding the discomfort of menstrual changes.

Chapter 7

Stress and the Risk of Cardiovascular Disorders Through a Type A Personality

Observation of cardiology cases in the 1950s convinced Friedman and Rosenman (1959) that patients with coronary heart disease frequently exhibited a common core of characteristics that became known as "Type A" or "Pattern A" behavior. Type A characteristics were thought to promote stress; the effects of stress somehow predisposed the individual to cardiovascular problems. By common agreement among researchers and practitioners, the Type A designation has been retained for the stress-promoting personality pattern, and individuals lacking such behaviors are identified as Type Bs. There have been sporadic complaints about this crude either-or typology, often centering upon the need for additional categories to allow for degrees of this personality style and the stress it promotes. In the main, however, the simple distinction between being a Type A or Type B personality has satisfied the researcher and the consumers of research alike.

Type A Behavior, Stress, and Cardiovascular Disorder

Type A behavior and stress. Friedman and Rosenman's (1959) early report of epidemiological evidence from a large study of presumably healthy men revealed that those who exhibited the Type A pattern were at several times the risk of coronary problems than were Type Bs. Their version of the Type A pattern included six behaviors: (1) An intense and continuing drive to attain personal goals which were frequently poorly defined, (2) extreme competitiveness, (3) persistent need for recognition and advancement, (4) accelerated rate of physical and mental functioning, (5) mental and physical alertness, and (6) continuous involvement in activities subject to time limits.

Although the general sense of the original Type A pattern has remained intact over the years, there have been numerous efforts to revise its components by deleting some behaviors or adding others. As an example of one such effort, Matthews (1982) described the Type A as demonstrating explosive and accelerated speech, concentrating on several things at once, dissatisfied with life, evaluating value in terms of numbers, prone to competing even in noncompetitional situations, and generally hostile. While this aggregate of characteristics seems to differ in several ways from those originally proposed, the disparity seems to evolve largely from Matthews' emphasis upon the ways in which underlying personality characteristics show themselves in discrete moment-to-moment behavior -- speech patterns, distracted concentration, devotion to numerical counts.

Friedman and Rosenman (1974) themselves eventually revised their concept of the Type A to emphasize extreme aggressiveness, hostility, time-urgency, and competitive achievement striving. Their thumbnail sketch describes the Type A as "aggressively involved in a chronic, incessant struggle to achieve more and more in less and less time, and if required to do so, against the opposing efforts of other things or other persons" (p. 67). The version of Type A personality that guided our research efforts closely approximated the Friedman and Rosenman model.

I could go on with a far more detailed version of the Type A person, taking into account 35 years of conceptualization and inquiry by researchers. However, I do not think that conveying the basic idea of pattern A behavior requires that much explanation. The Type A individual personifies the pure essence of a competitive society that holds out the promise of success to those who are willing to make the commitment and sacrifice necessary to outperform others. Being a Type A, however, sets the person apart from the mainstream achiever, although the difference is one of degree and not of kind. Each Type A component contributes in a functional sense to this extraordinary pattern. Being aggressive, even hostile, can open your way toward goals coveted by many but available to few; concern about competitors, implicit in humane qualities like warmth and sympathy, would only hold you back. Using time to good advantage is a plus to those seeking success. It is only the inability to tolerate a wasted moment or a temporarily slower pace that keeps the Type A constantly on edge and unable to relax. Competitive achievement striving is the centerpiece of the American success ethic and a virtue in the eyes of most who have sought or intend to seek distinction in their lives. Ultracompetitive Type As not only pit themselves against others in situations where winning and losing are critical to determining who is progressing, but they seek out existing competitive situations elsewhere if opportunities are otherwise lacking. They will even create competition if their search proves futile. To describe the Type A as obsessed with competition and success sounds a bit clinical for people who are still functioning within normal limits, but it does not miss the mark very far.

The dynamic importance of stress as a mediator of pathology has been presumed since the earliest descriptions of the Type A pattern and its proposed role in eventual coronary heart disease. The behaviors involved in the Type A's insatiable quest for achievement through competition, as well as those that constitute other components of the pattern, are not in themselves directly conducive to cardiovascular problems. If they were, many more of us would run the risk of heart disease. The emotions of stress, on the other hand, can disrupt cardiovascular integrity if they are strong enough and persist long enough. Hostility, which has attracted increasing attention as a Type A component, represents an exception to this set of observations. It is both an explicit component of the Type A pattern and one of the emotions of stress.

Perhaps because stress seemed to be such an obvious by-product of a Type A personality, it has been methodologically ignored in a great deal of Type A research. Treating stress as an inevitable consequence of Type A status, however defined, qualifies as a serious oversight when considering cardiovascular risk. At least, my research experience has taught me that when subjects under study are young and ambitious college students, the assumption that all Type As are seriously stressed can be readily dismissed. Some who show the behavioral pattern look very much like Type Bs as far as stress is concerned, although this will depend, of course, on how narrowly Type A status is defined. Identifying Type As by a mid-point split on a scale measuring this pattern likely would include many more who do not experience exceptional stress than would be true if a more extreme quartile split was employed.

My point here is that within an at-risk research methodology the definition of Type A status should include two safeguards before it can be considered anything close to ideal as a marker of cardiovascular risk. First of all, the Type A measure should be demonstrably sensitive to the arousal of stress; the behaviors described by the items ought to be those that are generally stress provoking. In addition, Type A measurement should be accompanied by an independent metric of stress level. Any measurement slippage in gauging Type A status as a precursor to a stress-related disorder would be compensated by the verification of a companion stress measure. By using both measures to identify critical Type A subjects, a researcher can be more confident that Type A status provokes enough stress to place someone at coronary risk.

Stress and cardiovascular disorder. The physiology of stress and its impact upon the cardiovascular system is not perfectly understood, although overview of the research (e.g., Price, 1982) clearly suggests that stress can produce varied and serious effects upon the heart, the vascular network, or blood functions. Any or all of these cardiovascular anomalies will be denoted by the term "coronary heart disease" (CHD) with the effects ranging from direct insult to the heart, through sclerotic changes in vascular walls, to elevated blood pressure or cholesterol count.

Reduced to simple terms, stress provides a risk to cardiovascular health in this way. A stressor evokes two types of response; a mental representation involves perception of some threat, and an emotional response follows more or less automatically when danger is perceived. Emotions triggered by perceived threat, whether they are experienced as fear, anger, jealousy, disgust, sadness, or another affect, activate the autonomic nervous system. The autonomic nervous system, in turn, initiates a release of substances into the blood stream from body organs. The substances, norepinephrine and epinephrine, have widespread biological effects that are thought to prepare the individual for "flight or fight." A major share of the changes instigated by the release of these substances is within the cardiovascular system. Paramount among these changes is the constriction of blood vessels. Vasoconstriction elevates blood pressure, and the heart must increase its workload in order to circulate blood and meet the body requirements for extra oxygen. At the same time, fatty acids are released into the blood, perhaps in preparation for an emergency, leading to elevated cholesterol.

Changes induced by activation of the autonomic nervous system during stress may have contributed to survival in the course of human evolution, and they may continue to prove adaptive on occasions even today. Furthermore, the biological impact of these natural responses is clearly tolerable given only periodic exposure to a stressor. Problems may arise, however, when a person is faced with chronic stress and the autonomic nervous system approaches a state of continuous activation. What begin as natural and self-protective reactions of the cardiovascular system to emergencies may challenge the limits of biological tolerance over time and introduce the risk of CHD.

    Type A research and assumptions regarding achievement. I cannot end these introductory remarks concerning Type A personality and the risk of stress-related CHD without commenting upon the immediate relevance of achievement-striving and competitiveness in this phase of our research. The role of these variables has been central to the theoretical framework for all of our stress-and-disorder investigations with college women, but up to this point thwarted ambition as a source of stress and symptom development has been a matter of judgment and not directly subjected to study. Women who fell short in their progress toward career and social goals and were less prepared for competition were thought to shift their achievement priorities to the attainment of a thin body and to place themselves at anorectic risk. That masculine women with contemporary values experienced increased menstrual and premenstrual distress was explained in part because of their sensitivity to and intolerance of changes within the reproductive cycle. Such changes would serve only as distractions from their predominant interest in successful career attainment. Feminine college women with traditional values must contend with stressful role conflict in which success in a career is viewed as incompatible with a desirable marriage and family.

    Now rather than depending upon what appear to be reasonable conclusions regarding the cost of ambition in some college women, our research will deal with achievement-striving and competitiveness directly. What required assumption before will be put to direct test as we consider whether the Type A pattern, as an aberration of competitive goal-seeking, qualifies as a convincing risk factor for cardiovascular disorder. In other words, this body of Type A evidence can be considered not only a test of the importance of the Type A personality pattern as a CHD risk factor but also a test of the achievement/competition assumptions in stress-related disorders.

Methodological Considerations Specific to Studying Type A Risk

    Subjects. The restriction of our at-risk Type A research to college students qualifies as advantageous for the most part, since it is difficult to imagine a better source of success-oriented, competitive women than the late-adolescents and young adults pursuing a higher education. While everyone within college ranks is not consumed by personal ambition, where else can you find such numbers of people with lofty career and interpersonal goals and the willingness to compete with others for their attainment? Given this subject pool, it is important to keep in mind that the crude dichotomy of subjects within each study, in which someone is either Type A or Type B, creates a difficult type of comparison. Type Bs, who serve as controls in our search for specific risk factors associated with Type A status, are themselves likely to be on the competitive and success-oriented side by general population standards. It is likely that the evidence from our Type A research would have turned out to be even more formidable if the controls had been easy-going replicas of the Type B prototype selected from a non-college population.

The investigation of Type A risk factors in CHD allowed me to address an important question that could not be considered in the other programs of risk research. Do the risk factors for stress-related psychobiological disorder in women differ in any important way from those that might be disclosed for men? Anorexia nervosa is a disorder that is found almost exclusively in females, and it would have been logistically impossible for me to generate groups of at-risk men for comparison. Disorders of the menstrual cycle are exclusive to women, of course. The appropriateness of Type A and Type B personality categories for predicting cardiovascular problems has been demonstrated for both sexes, although the bulk of research has been directed toward males. Many years ago, for example, Haynes, Feinleib, and Kannel (1980) reported that Type A working women are twice as likely to show heart problems than Type B working women. When they considered housewives, three times as many Type As suffered some form of CHD as Type Bs.

Given the relevance of Type A status to future CHD for both women and men, we were offered the opportunity to consider risk across gender. Do the same indicators of vulnerability found for women also emerge for men, and do these risk factors foretell greater vulnerability for one gender or the other? Sometimes the gender comparisons will be handled by preliminary analysis as a prelude to combining data across sexes for greater reliability if no differences are found. At other times, the results will be reported separately by sex. In either case, gender equivalence or disparity will receive comment. The sum of evidence will cast light not only on Type A women and their risk of stress-related CHD but upon whether female risk factors are distinct from those facing Type A men. To the extent that college women and college men present the same results, the gender comparisons provide an added bonus. Replication across sex should increase our confidence in whatever the evidence might be.

Type A measurement. The evolution of measurement within the Type A field of research involved a shift from the costly interview-based assessment procedures used in the influential Western Collaborative Group Study (Rosenman, Friedman, & Straus, 1964; Rosenman, Friedman, Straus, Wurm, Jenkins, & Messinger, 1966) to the more time-efficient and staff-conserving self-report questionnaire that subsequently gained popularity. The structured interview, the Type A measure of choice in this pioneer study, involved a number of questions put directly to subjects concerning their characteristic ways of dealing with situations capable of eliciting impatience, hostility, and competitiveness. The substance of the subject's answers to these questions contributed to identifying the Type A, but formal features of interview behavior, particularly speech, were given even greater priority in reaching this judgment. Whether the subject demonstrated pressured speech, interrupted the interviewer, filled in gaps of silence, acted with impatience or annoyance, etc., were used as stylistic indicators of Type A status. Observations of style in the interview were combined with substantive evidence of Type A behaviors taken from the subject's report of daily conduct to reach a summary judgment.

It became clear within the Western Collaborative Group Study research team that the logistical cost of the structured interview was too high even though it did allow Type A estimates that contributed to CHD prediction (Caffrey, 1970; Keith, Lown, & Stare, 1965; Rosenman et al., 1964). These Type A experts, most notably Jenkins (Jenkins, Rosenman, & Zyzanski, 1974; Jenkins, Zyzanski, & Rosenman, 1971; Jenkins, Zyzanski, Rosenman, & Cleveland, 1971; Kenigsberg, Zyzanski, Jenkins, Wardwell, & Licciardello, 1974), developed a self-report questionnaire to be completed by the subject. This inventory was intended to be a quicker, less expensive, more uniform, and better calibrated procedure for assessing Type A behavior on a group basis.

Initial validation of the Jenkins Activity Survey (JAS) was achieved by a 72% agreement rate with the structured interview, and this was followed by encouraging evidence of its validity for predicting CHD (see

Jenkins' references above). Despite this encouraging start, limitations shared with all self-report personality questionnaires soon became evident. Negative studies using the JAS were reported in which expected contingencies between Type A status and cardiovascular defect failed to materialize (Blumenthal, Williams, Kong, Schanberg & Thompson, 1978; Case, Heller, Case, Moss, & the Multicenter Post-infarction Research Group, 1985; Dimsdale, Hackett, Hutter, Block, & Catanzano, 1978; Dimsdale, Hackett, Hutter, Block, Catanzano, & White, 1979). It was not clear whether the inconsistent psychometric evidence should be blamed upon basic Type A theory, the specific components of Type A personality emphasized by the JAS, or upon exclusive use of subject self-report for information.

The popularity of the JAS in Type A research, along with other self-report scales purporting to measure the Type A construct, is a matter of record. In my opinion, however, the ready acceptance of these Type A scales brought dwindling progress to Type A research, but for a reason that received little notice from a generation of researchers. As I suggested earlier in this chapter, given the way that the Type A pattern of behavior is conceptualized, it is tempting to conclude that any person reporting that pattern will automatically experience a heavy stress load. Given hard-driving achievement-striving, a competitive nature, time-urgency, and hostile affect, the person must inevitably suffer the fate of high stress, or so it would seem.

What if this assumption of stress provocation for the Type A pattern leads to serious overgeneralization? While the Type A pattern of behavior must certainly be accepted as emotionally evocative, there may be many who are able to maintain Type A behaviors without exceptional stress. These "false-positive" Type As, assumed to be under serious stress when they are not, would certainly curtail the prediction of CHD if they were included with their stressed counterparts. Negative outcomes would be more likely. These false positives would also confound the effort to identify additional risk factors for CHD using our methodology, since the search is based upon the assumption that vulnerability derives from stress induced by Type A behaviors.

The concern over whether our Type A measure of choice properly identified subjects under serious stress led me to seek a psychometric procedure that would offer a better guarantee of accomplishing this end (see below). In addition, many of the Type A studies to be reported in forthcoming chapters will have used an additional precaution. By introducing an independent stress measure into these studies, stress-prone Type As could be isolated by psychometrically filtering the subjects twice. Those who have been identified as Type A by a scale devised as sensitive to stress level would then be authenticated as being under high stress by an independent scale before they were identified as the critical risk group. This cautious approach to identifying at-risk Type As also spun off a new kind of control group for comparisons beyond the usual Type B -- the person who manages Type A behavior without experiencing much stress.

Heilbrun, Palchanis, and Friedberg (1986) considered the Type A measurement problem created by the uncertainty of stress level associated with high scores. We examined the JAS, as a popular Type A measure, to determine if a more refined scale best suited for college students could be developed from among its items that would better insure the Type A would be highly stressed. Two studies bearing upon scale revision reported in this 1986 paper will be discussed at this point. The initial study considered a factor analysis involving the 44 items on the college form of the JAS along with the 25 stress symptoms from the checklist routinely included in our research. Factor analysis, simply stated, is a statistical procedure in which the correlations between responses to included items are processed statistically to determine which item responses tend to cluster together. The groupings of associated items are called "factors," and these derive meaning by examination of item content. The analysis may identify a variable number of factors depending upon how subjects respond to the items as well as upon other technical considerations.

Almost 200 undergraduates, roughly divided by sex, were administered the JAS and stress-rating forms. Their responses were subjected to factor analysis to determine whether there might be a subset of JAS items that clustered with stress symptoms and others that bore no relationship to stress. Only one factor emerged from the factor analysis. It contained 12 JAS items and 24 out of the 25 stress symptoms. These results seem quite compelling. Subjects who tended to endorse these 12 Type A items also tended to report a wide range of stress symptoms. Responses to the remaining 32 JAS items were unrelated to stress.

The JAS items that proved to be stress-related described three kinds of Type A behaviors. Two of these -- an urgent need to fill time with activity and a hard-driving and competitive nature -- are the essence of achievement-striving in the college student, and the third was hostile/irritable affect. Though the number of stress-related items was not large, they covered the basic core of the original Type A construct. The 12 JAS items were proposed as a special stress-prone Type A scale which, if used, would better guarantee that college students identified by higher scores as Type A would also experience high stress. We came to rely on this scale in our Type A research, although we always administered the complete JAS college form in order to retain the standardized context for the critical items. As I have said, an independent measure of stress also was included in most studies in order to more fully guarantee that our Type A college students experienced the stress required to put them at risk for CHD.

The second study described in the Heilbrun, Palchanis, and Friedberg (1986) paper represented an effort to confirm the implications of the factor analysis. A new sample of about 100 college subjects, half males and half females, was given the 44-item college form of the JAS along with the stress-symptom rating scales. The purpose of this study was to determine the correlation between the special (stress-prone) Type A scale and rated stress and to compare this figure with correlations generated by other item combinations from the parent JAS questionnaire. The special 12-item Type A scale was scored by assigning the highest score on an item to the multiple-choice option corresponding to the basic Type A construct. Other item combinations were assigned scores by keying the clearest Type A alternatives or other behaviors describing exceptional degrees of activity. Decreasing score values were assigned to options on all items as they departed more and more from the keyed alternative.

The results of the second study confirmed the value of the special Type A scale. Scores on this scale correlated .50 ($p < .005$) with the stress score for females and .43 ($p < .005$) with stress for males. These correlations are high enough to show that Type As identified by the special scale would likely be under stress. Yet they were not so high as to suggest redundancy and to preclude the value of further assistance from an independent stress measure to weed out psychometric errors. Other correlations between item combinations and stress stand in contrast to those produced by the special Type A scale. The standard Type A scale scored from the JAS provided the same negligible correlation with the stress measure ($r = .08$) for both males and females. Much the same result was obtained when the 32 JAS items left over from the 12-

item scale were correlated with stress. The relationships for females ($r = .04$) and males ($r = .07$) were next to nothing. These results, along with those found in the first factor-analysis study, substantiate my concern about whether standard questionnaire versions of Type A status should be used for assessing CHD risk without some further confirmation of stress.

Strategy of research. The strategy of investigation in anorectic and menstrual risk research reported earlier turned out to be straightforward enough. Risk factors in anorexia nervosa, including stress that would serve to motivate change, were largely to be found in those cognitive or social variables that would be conducive to any of three things. A personal characteristic might interfere with competitive achievement, promote the desire for a thin body, or assist the woman in restraining her eating behavior. Distinct from this, risk factors in disorders of the menstrual cycle appeared to contribute in two ways. They could increase the woman's sensitivity to the menstrual changes that she regularly experiences or introduce additional stress effects that become part of premenstrual or menstrual discomfort. These categorizations contributed to research strategies, since they helped me to select which variables held promise for investigation and to guide how interpretation of evidence should proceed.

In the case of Type A status and future risk of CHD, yet another strategy of search for additional risk factors seemed in order. One concern, as I hope was made evident earlier in this chapter, was that being a Type A would in itself present a danger of future cardiovascular disorder only if the behaviors contributed to higher stress levels. The search for Type A risk factors placed heavy emphasis upon traits that would promote stress in a Type A college student. However, even heavy stress would not introduce a convincing threat of CHD if observed at a young age. Being 18 years old, Type A, and under stress does not automatically translate into being at-risk years later when cardiovascular problems are more likely to appear. The age-relevance of our research findings became our second concern. It became necessary to go beyond the usual assumption of stability for personality characteristics (e.g., Once a Type A, always a Type A) and to identify traits (or their absence) that could account for an extended period of risk.

In answer to both concerns, the actuality of present stress in the Type A and her continued risk into later years, we conceived of risk factors as functioning in one of three ways in promoting stress. Two of these functional categories were viewed as more critical to current stress and the third as being especially relevant to prolonging vulnerability. Some traits might add to the Type A stress load by serving as additional sources of <u>arousal</u>. Other traits might make the burden of stress even worse by <u>augmenting</u> the amount of stress once it is aroused. A third set of traits could contribute to risk by making it more likely that stress would be <u>maintained</u> over longer time intervals. The personality characteristics fostering arousal and augmentation of stress can be recognized as relevant to current stress levels, whereas those contributing to maintaining stress would help explain the chronicity required for eventual breakdown of cardiovascular functions.

Chapter 8

Type A Behavior, Stress and the Risk of Cardiovascular Disorders: Specific Risk Factors Related to Arousal

The origins of CHD risk in Type A status seem logical enough. Given a Type A personality, the woman is hypercompetitive in situations that call for competition and in other situations that do not. The remaining attributes basic to the Type A pattern -- aggressive, hostile, time-urgent, hard-driving, and achievement striving (Rosenman, 1978) -- serve to motivate and shape competitive behavior to a fine edge. The Type A competitive lifestyle would be expected to generate considerable stress as the woman routinely interjects herself into contests where winning or losing are at stake. Given elevated and continuing stress, the chronic activation of the autonomic nervous system can have damaging effects upon the cardiovascular system.

Being competitive and under stress does not set the Type A college student that far apart from her peers who are themselves motivated for success and, to a variable extent, committed to competition for long-range goals. To distinguish the Type A who is at-risk for stress-related CHD years down the line, it seemed crucial to further elaborate a risk pattern. Cognitive and social personality traits not traditionally included in the Type A pattern had to be discovered as a basis for predicting future cardiovascular risk. These specific risk factors, when considered in combination with Type A status, should account for higher stress burdens than shown by Type Bs. Even more critical, these specific factors should allow the more difficult discrimination in stress level from other Type As who lack these risk-conferring traits. These specific factors also should offer some explanation for the chronicity of stress required before the cardiovascular system would be expected to capitulate.

The research strategy for bringing CHD risk into finer focus for the Type A college student will be familiar to the reader. Women (and men) will be subdivided by the relative presence or absence of a Type A personality pattern, and these groupings will be assessed for level of everyday stress after being further broken down by the strength of additional risk factors. The assignment of these factors to particular functional risk categories comes down to my personal judgment. Accordingly, the categories of risk variables -- those that appear to influence arousal, augmentation, or maintenance of stress -- are subject to overlap and revision. I recognize that in my effort to make stress effects more understandable I may have oversimplified the idea of how behaviors contribute to the stress experienced by the Type A. A personality trait could increase stress problems in more than one way, perhaps in all three. Allow me to use self-control as a case in point, since it is to be included in this chapter on factors relating to stress arousal in the at-risk Type A.

I conceived of self-control as falling in the stress-arousal category, since diminished self-control could readily expand the range of situations in which the Type A woman is required to compete like everyone else, seeks out competition, or even introduces competition where none otherwise exists. Since competition evokes some degree of stress for most people, the more opportunities for competing, the greater the amount of stress aroused by competition. At the same time, limited self-control could make matters worse once the Type A enters a stress-arousing competitive situation. Augmentation of expected stress could result from a poor containment of competitive behaviors that turn the most insignificant competition into a major contest. Finally, poor self-control could nourish stress over time as the Type A woman is unable to restrain her stress-provoking competitive ways despite awareness of their cost. I could have considered self-control as part of any of these risk categories. It should be noted, however, that no matter how imperfect the categorization, validation will still be gauged by a significant elevation in stress as the risk factor is paired with Type A status.

Self-control as a Specific Risk Factor for Coronary-prone Type As

Heilbrun and Friedberg (1988) explored the role of self-control in determining stress level in Type A women and men. Interest in self-control as a risk factor, as explained before, was predicated primarily upon the Type A's tendency to compete in not only the usual ways open to college students but to seek out or even create opportunities for competition in other situations. For the Type A woman who lacks self-control, this readiness for competition could be pervasive enough to arouse excessive stress. In addition, deficits in self-control could have stressful consequences as competitive situations are allowed to get out of hand or the woman fails to restrain her ultracompetitive ways over time despite the problems they create. Type As with better self-control should be in a position to restrict their competitive urge and to spare themselves the cost of excessive involvement.

This investigation included 82 college subjects, split evenly by sex. The self-control battery was described in an earlier chapter as the basis for comparing the cognitive underpinnings of self-regulation in women at-risk for bulimia and anorexia nervosa (Heilbrun & Bloomfield, 1986). It may be recalled that the standard laboratory battery includes: (1) two measures of impulse control, (2) two tasks gauging how broadly the person responds to information, thereby making it more likely that alternatives to impulsive response will be available (reflectiveness); and (3) a task estimating self-reinforcement effectiveness, the extent to which the person can influence her own intended behavior by positive or negative personal evaluation. Time restraints prevented the inclusion of the self-reinforment measure in the Heilbrun and Bloomfield study, but all five laboratory tasks were included in the Heilbrun and Friedberg investigation.

Self-control, as before, was approached as a complex skill involving several cognitive functions. The index of self-control was a composite of the five discrete scores after each was transformed to the same standard score distribution ($M = 50$, $\underline{SD} = 10$). Our stress measure was the familiar symptom-rating procedure that asked the subjects to rate the prevalence of 25 stress indicators over the previous year. Type A and B status were determined by the sample median on the special 12-item JAS scale that includes only stress-related Type A behaviors.

Analysis proceeded by stages in order to answer several questions regarding self-control and Type A risk. The preliminary analysis concerned whether Type As were generally less capable of self-control than Type Bs and whether this depended upon the sex of the subject?

Results relevant to this analysis are found in Table 8.1. Perhaps the most obvious thing about these composite self-control scores is that they show opposite patterns for the two sexes, and a significant (p < .01) interaction effect verified that impression. Female Type As demonstrated superior self-control when compared to Type B controls (p < .05); the reverse effect was observed for male Type As whose self-control was inferior to Type B males (p < .05).

Women college students did not provide the preliminary results that had been expected. Female Type As were more capable of self-control than their Type B peers. The logical expectation that Type As would generally lack restraint as they revert to competition, fill their time with activity, and express hostile/irritable affect was not accommodated by these findings. Given the first opportunity to compare college women with college men, we already find a difference in the Type A domain, since the male subjects did conform to expectation as far as self-control and Type A behavior were concerned. Competitive excesses suggested by the Type A behavioral pattern did occur in concert with less self-control for college men.

The unexpected interaction between Type A/B and gender in degree of self-control raises an intriguing question regarding the common-ground between Type A behaviors and the instrumental (goal-oriented) qualities of the traditional masculine role. These are certainly not identical patterns, but there are important overlapping features. Both entail being competitive, achievement-striving, and aggressive for examples. This suggests that the interaction involving Type A/B status, self-control and gender may have much to do with lingering social pressure. Men must still contend with traditional expectations that would have them compete and achieve by whatever aggressive means they have at their disposal. College women who subscribe to traditional male expectations, including aggressive competition for success, might well confront lingering opposition to their choice or, at least, perceive opposition to be present. In order to defy the legacy of traditional role expectations, Type A women may have to fall back on superior self-control. Type B college men could be in much the same situation as they resist falling in line with "hard-charging" expectations for their sex.

The next analysis brings us to whether self-control capabilities can be considered a specific CHD risk factor in Type A college students and whether gender again plays a role. This issue was evaluated by splitting Type A and Type B females into those with better and poorer self-

Table 8.1.   Self-control Capabilities[a] for Type A and Type B College Students

	Females				Males			
	Type A		Type B		Type A		Type B	
N	M	N	M	N	M	N	M
21	260.96	21	244.74	19	238.32	21	255.24

[a]Scores for all five self-control measures were transformed into standard scores with a mean of 50 and standard deviation of 10 before combining them into composite self-control scores for each subject. Higher scores indicate better self-control.

Note. - Adapted from Heilbrun, A. B., & Friedberg, E. B. (1988). Type A, self-control, and vulnerability to stress. Journal of Personality Assessment, 52, 420-433.

control (defined by composite score for the entire sample median) and examining the levels of stress reported by each group. Males were distributed in the same way. Preliminary analysis of stress results separately by sex revealed no hint of a gender difference; whatever relationships were revealed held equally true for women and men. Accordingly, sexes were combined in order to generate larger and more stable groups. Table 8.2 includes the stress reported by Type A and B college students who demonstrate relative superior and inferior self-control.

Statistical analysis of the Table 8.2 results revealed the expected elevation in stress scores for Type As relative to Type Bs ($p < .01$). This expected overall effect affirms the success of our revised Type A scale in capturing the required essence of the construct -- a pattern of behaviors that promote stress and put the person at general risk for CHD. Only one group was responsible for this effect, however. Lack of self-control in Type As, whether they were women or men, was associated with extraordinarily high stress, far beyond the stress level reported by any other group ($ps < .001$). Type As with better self-control did not differ in stress level from either low-stress Type B group. As I have emphasized in preliminary remarks concerning research methodology, simply being Type A, as we categorically defined such status, was not in itself an open invitation to burgeoning stress. Given better self-control, the Type As in our sample looked very much like their less competitive Type B peers.

Despite the fact that the preliminary analysis found female Type As more gifted in self-control than male Type As, the nature of specific risk was the same for both sexes. Despite being fewer in number, Type A college women with weaker self-control suffered higher stress; the more commonplace association between Type A status and poor self-control in college men also resulted in elevated stress. Though the dynamics of risk, as far as they involve self-control, are at some variance when women are compared to men, the end result appears to be the same. Poor self-control lends CHD risk to being a Type A by its association with elevated stress.

Locus of Control of Reinforcement as a Specific Risk Factor for Coronary-prone Type As

Just as cognitive limitations may decrease the at-risk Type A woman's actual control over her behavior and open the way to poorly

Table 8.2.   Stress Reported by Type A and Type B College Students Varying in Self-control

Level of Self-control	Type A		Type B	
	$\underline{N}$[a]	$\underline{M}$	$\underline{N}$[a]	$\underline{M}$
Better	21	40.90	28	35.78
Poorer	19	55.89	24	36.79

[a]The composition by sex was: Type A/better self-control, 14 women and 7 men; Type A/poorer self-control, 7 women and 12 men; Type B/better self-control, 6 women and 12 men; Type B/poorer self-control, 15 women and 9 men.

Note. - Adapted from Heilbrun, A. B., & Friedberg, E. B. (1988). Type A., self-control, and vulnerability to stress. Journal of Personality Assessment, 52, 420-433.

governed competitiveness and frequent arousal of stress across an expanse of situations, a limited sense of control over reinforcement outcomes appears capable of much the same effect. This reasoning led to an investigation (Heilbrun, 1989) of stress-vulnerability in Type As considered further by locus of control of reinforcement (LOC). LOC, an attitudinal variable attributed to Rotter (1966), has attracted an incredible amount of research, perhaps because it appeals so readily to common sense. This construct refers to the person's general expectation that the consequences of her actions are determined by the nature of those actions or are determined by outside forces.

An external locus of control represents the view held by a person that whatever she does, the reinforcement (reward or punishment) will depend upon forces beyond the control of that individual -- important others, luck, chance, fate, destiny, whatever. An internal locus of control refers to the person's belief that she determines and is responsible for reinforcement outcomes, whether things turn out well or badly. Being external or internal in orientation is rarely, if ever, a matter of being committed to such absolute extremes. Rather, individual differences exist in the relative degree to which people maintain these two attitudes. For sake of convenience, research samples are often dichotomized into external and internal types, just as researchers subdivide samples into Type A and Type B. LOC types are best understood, then, as relative groupings in which people generally lack a sense of personal control over how their actions will be reinforced (externals) or generally feel that their own actions will determine whether reinforcements turn out to be negative or positive (internals).

I anticipated that an external LOC in the competitive Type A would promote stress for at least two reasons. For one, being competitive and ambitious does not guarantee coming out ahead in the win/lose contests courted so avidly by the at-risk Type A. Sheer competition arouses the emotions of stress but so does the prospect of losing, especially in someone so committed to besting others. If the Type A woman has experienced her share of failure in past competitive situations, experience should serve as a realistic source of restraint. However, if the Type A woman were also external, the restraint derived from past reality might be lost. After all, the next competitive adventure could very well turn out better than past failures, since previous competitive outcomes are not thought to be contingent upon her own behaviors.

Not only might externality contribute to stress in the Type A by compromising competitive restraint based upon previous experience, an arousal effect, but an external LOC could result in extra stress within each competitive situation, an augmenting effect. The external Type A enters into competition, where winning or losing really matters, lacking the sense that her own actions will determine whether she is victor or vanquished. This might contribute to a fatalistic calm in some. More likely, it would promote a sense of helplessness and dismay in the woman dedicated to achievement by outperforming others, a seemingly sure-fire way to increase the stress of competition.

Heilbrun's (1989) study of the interface between Type A/B stand-ing, LOC, and stress involved the usual 12-item JAS Type A scale and stress-symptom ratings along with the Adult Nowicki-Strickland Internal-External Locus of Control scale (Nowicki & Duke, 1974). The 120 college subjects were split evenly by gender. In this study preliminary analysis revealed that the relationships were comparable for both sexes, so subjects were combined over gender for the final stress analysis. It also appeared obvious by inspection that Type A/B status was unrelated to LOC; Type As of either sex were not inclined to be external or internal, and the same was true for Type Bs.

Average stress scores were determined for the four subgroups formed by splitting the sample distributions on the Type A and LOC measures at their respective medians. Table 8.3 presents these mean figures. Statistical analysis disclosed the expected powerful effect of Type A status ($p < .001$) along with a significant effect of externality ($p < .05$). Each effect had its origins in the remarkably elevated stress scores of Type A externals. The stress reported by Type A externals exceeded that of any other group (all $ps < .001$). Stress ratings of Type A internals did not differ statistically from external or internal Type Bs. LOC within Type B college students did not distinguish in a reliable way between those who were more and less stressed; externality was a specific risk factor only if it appeared in a Type A.

The LOC results were clearcut. Type A women, lacking in the sense of controlling their own reinforced outcomes, show a singular elevation in stress and the greatest risk for CHD. Male external Type As, indistinguishable from their female counterparts with whom they were combined in the analysis, also reported a uniquely high stress level and revealed themselves to be at highest CHD risk.

Table 8.3.   Level of Stress reported by Type A and Type B College Students Differing in Locus of Control

Locus of Control	Type A		Type B	
	$\underline{N}$	$\underline{M}$	$\underline{N}$	$\underline{M}$
External	31	57.68	30	38.33
Internal	30	40.60	29	32.14

Note. - Adapted from Heilbrun, A. B. (1989). Type A, locus of control, and stress: Another case in point. *Psychological Reports*, 64, 524-526.

Combined Risk of Limited Self-control and External Locus of Control in Type A Women

Independent studies had identified poorer self-control (Heilbrun & Friedberg, 1988) and an external locus of control (Heilbrun, 1989) as specific risk factors when found in Type A women (and Type A men). The question remained whether these two control factors actually contribute independently to stress level in the Type A, each adding to CHD vulnerability. The alternative of grossly overlapping stress effects for poor self-control and an external LOC would mean that the presence of both in company with the Type A pattern was no more risk-provoking than the presence of one. I collected a follow-up sample of 94 college women to consider that question. The battery of questionnaires included the special Type A scale on the JAS, the checklist of stress symptoms, and the Nowicki-Strickland LOC scale; a separate laboratory session was required to measure the cognitive underpinnings of self-control. This follow-up Type A study did not include males, since the agreement across gender of both self-control and LOC implications for CHD risk already was a matter of record.

Analysis of joint risk proceeded by determining Type A/Type B, external/ internal LOC, and better/poorer self-control in terms of the sample median on each distribution. Independent contributions of the two risk factors nominally allied with control were tested by constituting three risk groups and comparing their relative levels of stress. A high-risk group was made up of Type A women who displayed both poorer self-control and an external LOC. An intermediate group of Type As showed one but not the other specific risk factor, and low-risk Type As were defined by having neither factor in evidence. Type Bs were grouped by the same assignment rules for the two control factors. Table 8.4 includes the amount of life-stress reported by these six groups.

As Table 8.4 suggests, the presence of both specific risk factors in the Type A college woman resulted in a singularly high level of stress ($\underline{M} = 60.17$). This was far in excess of the stress reported by other Type As that displayed either limited self-control or an external LOC ($\underline{M} = 44.96$). In fact, the presence of one risk factor was accompanied by slightly less stress than was found in the Type A women who displayed neither risk factor ($\underline{M} = 47.80$). These Type A stress levels varied significantly ($\underline{p} < .01$), allowing for the conclusion that self-control deficit and an external LOC each contributes its own stress-arousing effects. In fact, without their combined presence, neither

Table 8.4.   Level of Stress Reported by Type A and Type B College Women Given the Presence of Poorer Self-control and an External LOC as Specific Risk Factors

	Type A			Type B		
	Both Risk Factors Present	Either Risk Factor Present	Neither Risk Factor Present	Both Risk Factors Present	Either Risk Factor Present	Neither Risk Factor Present
	$\underline{N}$ $\underline{M}$	$\underline{N}$ $\underline{M}$	$\underline{N}$ $\underline{M}$	$\underline{N}$ $\underline{M}$	$\underline{N}$ $\underline{M}$	$\underline{N}$ $\underline{M}$
	12 60.17	26 44.96	10 47.80	8 40.62	29 37.31	9 33.78

specific risk factor seemed to matter as far as stress was concerned. The average stress levels provided by these risk groupings for Type Bs were generally low (Ms = 33.78-40.62) and did not differ from each other statistically.

Again we can see radical differences in stress levels reported by Type A college women depending in this case upon the presence and incremental contributions of two risk factors. Some Type A women were shown to be at-risk because of very high stress, but even more of the Type As (75%) revealed nothing extraordinary in way of stress or CHD risk. Furthermore, the added provocation that the self-control and LOC variables contributed together to   CHD risk in Type A women was not evident in the Type B. Both requirements of risk analysis for isolating a specific effect within pattern A women were satisfied.

Sex-role Status as a Specific Risk Factor for Coronary-prone Type As

The sex-roles traditionally assigned to women and men in our culture qualified as important risk factors for the two stress-related disorders that have received attention in earlier chapters. The feminine woman was found to be more at-risk for anorexia nervosa, with the finding explained by her problems in competing for the usual targets of success and her more ready acceptance of body thinness as a substitute goal. Unadulterated masculinity and femininity were indicted as risk factors in menstrual-cycle disorders but for different reasons. Sensitivity to and lack of tolerance for menstrual changes were proposed as important for the masculine college woman whose contemporary attitudes were consonent with her sex-role behavior. The infusion of stress from role conflict and competition into the bodily disturbances provided by menstrual changes were thought to magnify symptoms for the feminine woman whose behavior and attitudes were traditional. Only college women reporting sex-role behaviors that were counterbalanced by opposing attitudes escaped menstrual and premenstrual dysfunction.

In approaching the possible relevance of sex-role commitment to Type A status and the risk of CHD, yet another dynamic possibility loomed as important. On an a priori basis, the masculine woman seemed most at-risk for CHD because of the behavioral overlap between the traditional role for men and the Type A pattern. The overlap with masculinity could lend itself to a more compelling Type A effect. I have alluded to the similarity between traditional masculinity, especially its instrumental core, and some aspects of the Type A pattern earlier in this chapter. Instrumental orientation within the traditional male sex-role emphasizes personal goal-seeking and doing whatever seems necessary to achieve your own ends, including offending others who stand in your way. This contrasts with the traditional feminine expressive orientation that emphasizes interpersonal harmony and the importance of giving to others in order to receive warmth in return.

The instrumental quality of egoistic goal-seeking bears a motivational similarity to the competitive, achievement-oriented, time-urgent inclinations of the Type A person. Risk for the masculine woman, given this similarity, would reside in the ease with which she could slide into excesses of striving and winning at any cost even for a Type A. With excess comes stress as the woman's masculine, instrumental nature is compounded by Type A competitive striving for achievement. The possibility that masculinity and Type A status might not compound their effects but simply be redundant behavior patterns also had to be considered.

Although many men do not relish the harsh qualities of masculinity, it still remains as a social expectation for males in many quarters. An examination of the male evidence promised an interesting look at whether masculinity serves as a specific risk factor for Type A men as seemed possible with women. The question with college men became whether the striving excesses of compounded instrumental and Type A behaviors would serve as a special source of stress even though the behaviors are more in line with traditional expectation for males?

The first paper considering sex-role and Type A/B personality (Heilbrun, Palchanis, & Friedberg, 1986) was centrally concerned with the development and validation of the special JAS Type A scale. Two studies reported in this paper and bearing upon scale development were discussed in the previous chapter. A third study described in the 1986 paper is relevant at this point. The third body of evidence considered whether a more elaborated pattern of personality correlates might be discovered for the Type A construct if stress-relevant Type A measurement was introduced. Dembroski (1978) had little success in extending the traits associated with being Type A using standard JAS measurement; availability of the new 12-item Type A scale encouraged another try.

The examination of sex-role status for stress-prone female and male Type As was among the focused concerns of this third study as was the level of maladjustment implicit in the elaborated personality profiles.

Prior studies into the sex-role status of Type As offered somewhat inconsistent results. Type As emerged as more masculine than Type Bs in several studies (Batlis & Small, 1982; DeGregorio & Carver, 1990; Nix & Lohr, 1981), although two of the three studies failed to find an accompanying deficit in femininity among Type As (DeGregorio & Carver, 1980; Nix & Lohr, 1981). None of these previous investigators, it might be pointed out, had used a Type A inventory with a demonstrated relevance to stress.

Heilbrun, Palchanis, and Friedberg used a sample of 51 females and 50 males from campus to search for extended personality correlates of Type A or Type B status. The subjects had completed the JAS along with the self-report Adjective Check List (Gough & Heilbrun, 1980), a compilation of 300 commonly-used behavioral adjectives. After dividing the females into Types A or B by median split on the special JAS scale, their rates for endorsement as self-characteristic were compared for each of the 300 traits. The same procedure was followed separately for the male subjects.

After using appropriate statistics to establish which personality characteristics distinguished Type A and Type B college women (and, independently, Type A and Type B college men), we determined the quality of these differentiating traits along sex-role and social-adaptation lines. This was made possible by the availability of sex-role stereotype and adjustment values for all 300 traits (Williams & Best, 1982) on the Adjective Check List. These normative values, based upon the judgments of college students, allowed us to discern whether stress-prone Type A women displayed the anticipated masculinity relative to Type Bs; by agreement among sex-role researchers, this required a pattern of high masculinity and low femininity. In addition, the norms indicating the social value of trait behaviors within our culture promised some insight into whether Type A behavior of the college woman is associated with a more general pattern of maladaptive personality traits that would be conducive to additional stress. Male Type A/B comparisons also were made as part of these qualitative analyses.

Tables 8.5 and 8.6 include the self-reported traits from the checklist that statistically distinguished Type A from Type B college students, presented separately by sex. The differentiating traits included those more commonly endorsed by Type As as well as traits that were less commonly observed in the Type A than the Type B. The sex-role and social-favorability values for college students are juxtaposed to each trait. Sex-role values greater than 500 are increasingly masculine, and

Table 8.5.   Personality Characteristics Distinguishing Stress-prone Type A from Type B College Females

	Stress-prone Type A More			Stress-prone Type A Less	
Trait	Sex-role Value	Adaptive Value	Trait	Sex-role Value	Adaptive Value
ambitious	702	599	affected	385	455
anxious	441	452	appreciative	317	618
argumentative	553	441	cheerful	343	641
cynical	558	403	discrete	423	560
deliberate	563	519	easygoing	577	604
demanding	567	453	gentle	312	635
faultfinding	452	379	hardhearted	597	372
hurried	446	437	imaginative	364	574
impatient	583	385	informal	576	552
impulsive	392	470	interests-wide	505	619
industrious	605	624	kind	374	645
opinionated	602	469	leisurely	515	529
outspoken	600	518	modest	411	569
quarrelsome	475	360	original	450	630
resentful	492	373	persevering	535	580
self-centered	561	353	reserved	464	511

Table 8.5 continued

| | Stress-prone Type A More | | | Stress-prone Type A Less | |
Trait	Sex-role Value	Adaptive Value	Trait	Sex-role Value	Adaptive Value
shrewd	522	498	sincere	403	630
sophisticated	402	549	spontaneous	466	553
temperamental	416	425	thoughtful	419	627
touchy	456	402	tolerant	446	598
tough	649	520	trusting	409	620
worrying	428	393	unselfish	440	622
			warm	341	640

Note. - Adapted from Heilbrun, A. B., Palchanis, N., & Friedberg, E. (1986). Self-report measurement of Type A behavior: Toward refinement and improved prediction. Journal of Personality Assessment, 50, 525-538.

Table 8.6.   Personality Characteristics Distinguishing Stress-prone Type A from Type B College Males

Trait	Stress-prone Type A More		Trait	Stress-prone Type A Less	
	Sex-role Value	Adaptive Value		Sex-role Value	Adaptive Value
ambitious	702	599	cool	601	535
anxious	441	452	cynical	538	403
cautious	398	551	forgetful	507	406
complaining	401	359	gentle	312	635
conservative	468	505	lazy	601	372
dependable	506	648	mischievous	596	464
determined	616	603	quiet	417	543
fair-minded	482	609	relaxed	530	604
greedy	576	343	unselfish	490	622
high-strung	379	439			
hurried	446	437			
impatient	583	385			
intolerant	579	375			
irritable	477	357			

Table 8.6 continued

Trait	Stress-prone Type A More		Stress-prone Type A Less
	Sex-role Value	Adaptive Value	
logical	661	599	
methodical	611	516	
quarrelsome	475	360	
serious	580	553	
stern	622	456	
tense	510	411	
touchy	456	402	
vindictive	503	399	
worrying	428	393	

Note. - Adapted from Heilbrun, A. B., Palchanis, N., & Friedberg, E. (1986). Self-report measurement of Type A behavior: Toward refinement and improved prediction. Journal of Personality Assessment, 50, 525-538.

those less than 500 become more feminine as values decrease. A more favorable adjustment for college students is represented by increasing values as they rise above 500, and unfavorable adjustment (with stress-provoking implications) is portrayed as values decrease below 500.

Preliminary analysis of the Adjective Check List personality traits that set Type A women and men apart from Type Bs considered whether agreement between the two self-report measures could be detected. We looked for two types of fit between the trait lists and the special JAS scale -- correspondence in terms of the components of the basic Type A pattern and correspondence in terms of the emotional impact of stress that would be expected given these Type A behaviors. Confidence in the self-report method requires some degree of agreement. I will not concern myself with whether correspondence results from traits in the women's list or the men's list; both contributed in about equal amounts.

Time-urgency in the Type A can be seen in the terms "hurried," "impatient," and being less "relaxed." Hostile and aggressive components within the Type A pattern are represented in traits like "complaining," "faultfinding," "intolerant," "irritable," "quarrelsome," "resentful," "tough," "vindictive," and less "gentle." The hard-driving and competitive nucleus of the Type A pattern is suggested by "ambitious," "determined," "industrious," and being less "easygoing," "leisurely," and "reserved." Emotional impact of stress is explicit in self-descriptions such as "anxious," "high-strung," "tense," "worrying," and less "relaxed" for the Type A.

These alignments reveal some degree of correspondence between the subjects' statements on the JAS and their selection of behavioral adjectives on the checklist, enough at least to assume consistency in describing their own behavior. For the most part though, the traits distinguishing Type A from Type B college students extended beyond the familiar core components of the coronary-prone pattern and the emotional impact of stress to include a broader array of personality attributes.

The sex-role quality of the terms in Tables 8.5 and 8.6 was analyzed by examining the pattern of traits setting the Type A and Type B student apart with respect to degree of conformity to traditional sex-role expectations. A sex-role deviance score was developed for female Type As by determining the algebraic deviation of Type A correlates from the normative middle value of 500. A plus or minus was assigned based upon whether the particular trait deviated in the masculine or feminine direction from 500 and whether it characterized the Type A by its relative presence or absence. For example, being "opinionated" for a college student received a value of 602 in the masculine direction. Since it was more characteristic of Type A than Type B women and represented deviance from sex-role stereotype, it received a deviance value of + 102 (602 - 500). "Appreciative" was relatively uncharacteristic of the Type A female relative to Type B and had a value of 317, portraying it as quite feminine. The absence of a feminine trait is as deviant as the presence of a masculine trait as far as conformity to stereotype is concerned, so the score assigned to this correlate of Type A status in women was + 183 (500 - 317). Minus deviance scores were assigned to Type A traits when Type A women were found to be better characterized by a feminine term or less aptly described by a masculine term. A counterpart scoring system was adopted to score sex-role deviance for Type A male characteristics.

The 45 traits representing Type A personality correlates for college women received an average sex-role deviance score of 42.07. In contrast, the 32 Type A correlates for the men averaged out at -9.62. These diverging means ($\underline{p} < .05$) portray female Type A traits as clearly deviating from traditional sex-role expectations, more masculine and less feminine than those of her Type B peer. The male Type A, however, varies little from the Type B when his personality correlates are examined. Given the negative values, even that small variation is in the direction of greater conformity to sex-role expectations for the personality correlates distinguishing Type A and Type B men.

A procedure for scoring degree of maladjustment for the personality features in Tables 8.5 and 8.6 involved a very similar set of rules. The procedure began by determining the arithmetic deviation of the adjustment score for each term from the normative mid-point of 500. Plus or minus values were assigned to these deviation scores in such a way as to reflect the quality of adjustment for Type A traits (relative to Type B). If a maladjustive trait (below 500) was present or an adjustive trait (above 500) was absent within the Type A list, a plus score was assigned. The presence of an adjustive characteristic or the absence of a maladjustive attribute resulted in the assignment of a minus value. The female Type A correlates received an average maladaptive value of 63.60, much higher than the 26.03 mean for the male Type A correlates ($\underline{p} < .05$).

Put the two sets of results together regarding the quality of Type A personality correlates, and the stress-prone Type A woman would be viewed as generally deviant from her Type B peers and excessively so relative to the same comparisons for men. She veers from traditional expectation in her sex-role behavior, being more masculine and less feminine than the Type B woman. At the same time, her distinguishing personality features bode poorly for her social adjustment. The Type A woman describes herself as argumentative, cynical, demanding, fault-finding, impatient, opinionated, quarrelsome, resentful, self-centered, touchy, and tough; these traits would hardly add to the effectiveness of her social relationships. This would be especially true, since they appear in her personality profile without compensating traits such as cheerful, gentle, kind, thoughtful, tolerant, and warm, displaced qualities that would mitigate the harshness of her interpersonal transactions. The masculine sex-role deviance leads me to expect a collaboration between an instrumental orientation and her Type A pattern. The dubious quality of her interpersonal transactions promises little social relief from her hard-charging ways. Both findings point toward a special problem with stress for the Type A college woman. The male Type A correlates did not suggest anything comparable with regard to sex-role deviance and adjustment.

Another effort to confirm the relationship between Type A standing and sex-role (Heilbrun, Wydra, & Friedberg, 1989) followed the 1986 investigation of personality correlates for the coronary-prone pattern. It seemed worthwhile to try to replicate the 1986 findings by a more conventional methodology (i.e., validated scales of masculinity and femininity) and to introduce the often-ignored gender-schema variable into the analysis to examine sex-role commitment from a second perspective. Gender-schema measurement allowed us to introduce a more refined version of sex-role into the risk picture by examining not only what the woman reports in way of sex-typed behavior but the extent to which she is sensitive to traditional sex-role expectations. Including two sex-role variables that often seem to be at variance within the same individual also made it possible to examine their almost unexplored interaction. In this case, the question became whether some combination of sex-role behavior and degree of sensitivity to traditional sex-role expectations would appear as part of the Type A pattern.

The 81 college subjects included in the Heilbrun, Wydra, and Friedberg (1989) study were split about evenly by sex. The JAS stress-prone Type A scale and stress-symptom questionnaire were used along with the laboratory task measuring gender schema, described earlier in the book. As a brief reminder, gender schema represents a cognitive organization that includes all information relevant to stereotyped sex-role behavior. Uninstructed memory for sex-typed information provides a yardstick of cognizance and sensitivity for traditional role behavior assigned to women and men. Finally, sex-role behavior was inferred from the Masculinity scale and Femininity scale (Heilbrun, 1976) scored from the Adjective Check List (Gough & Heilbrun, 1980). These sex-role scales, though less well-known than the more popular Bem (1974) and Spence, Helmreich, and Stapp (1975) instruments, work psychometrically about as effectively as either (Heilbrun, 1981; Kelly, Furman, & Young, 1978).

Comparisons in terms of masculinity and femininity were made for college subjects who fell into the Type A and Type B categories, as defined by the sample median Type A score. Table 8.7 includes the mean sex-role scores required for these comparisons. The Type A woman presented a sex-role pattern that showed her to be more masculine than feminine, whereas the Type B female revealed a level of femininity that exceeds her masculinity. An interaction effect ($\underline{p} < .05$) resulted. The results for females fell in line with the 1986 findings that showed the relative strength of the sex-role pattern for Type A women to lean toward predominant masculinity relative to her Type B peer. Male results led to the same conclusion reached by Heilbrun, Palchanis, and Friedberg (1986) as well; there are no sex-role distinctions between Type A and Type B college men.

Introduction of gender schema into the sex-role picture was accomplished by assigning Type A and B women to either a masculine group (masculinity score higher than femininity score) or a feminine group (femininity score higher than masculinity score). This arrangement of subjects was repeated for Type A and B men. Gender-schema scores for the resulting eight groups are presented in Table 8.8.

Reference to the Type A gender-schema scores in Table 8.8 reveals a wide discrepancy between female Type As once they are broken down into masculine and feminine groups ($\underline{p} < .01$), and the nature of the difference may come as a surprise. Masculine Type A females provided higher gender-schema scores ($\underline{M} = 42.92$) and feminine Type A women supplied lower gender-schema scores ($\underline{M} = 10.12$). In fact, as far as performance of college students on this laboratory task usually goes, the feminine Type A woman not only demonstrated lower scores in a relative sense but incredibly low scores in an absolute sense. This means that Type A females who are committed to nontraditional masculinity have remained sensitized to traditional sex-role expectations, whereas

Table 8.7.   Sex-role Characteristics Distinguishing Stress-prone Type A and Type B College Students

Sex-role Dimension	Females				Males			
	Type A ($\underline{N}$ = 20)		Type B ($\underline{N}$ = 20)		Type A ($\underline{N}$ = 20)		Type B ($\underline{N}$ = 21)	
	$\underline{M}$		$\underline{M}$		$\underline{M}$		$\underline{M}$	
Masculinity	56.20		47.10		51.35		50.48	
Femininity	50.80		51.15		46.10		47.62	

Note. - Adapted from Heilbrun, A. B., Wydra, D., & Friedberg, L. (1989). Sex role correlates of stress-prone Type A behavior in college students. Sex Roles, 21, 433-448.

Table 8.8.　　Gender-schema Scores for Masculine and Feminine Stress-prone Type A and Type B College Students

Gender	Type A				Type B			
	Masculine		Feminine		Masculine		Feminine	
	$\underline{N}$	$\underline{M}$	$\underline{N}$	$\underline{M}$	$\underline{N}$	$\underline{M}$	$\underline{N}$	$\underline{M}$
Females	12	42.92	8	10.12	8	37.12	12	45.92
Males	10	36.10	10	31.10	12	46.75	9	45.44

Note. - Adapted from Heilbrun, A. B., Wydra, D., & Friedberg, L. (1989). Sex role correlates of stress-prone Type A behavior in college students. Sex Roles, 21, 433-448.

traditional feminine Type A females have essentially lost touch with culturally-prescribed role boundaries between men and women . No gender-schema difference was noted between masculine and feminine Type B females, although the direction of difference at least returned the findings to a correspondence between traditional social behavior and sensitivity to traditional stereotypes. The overall interaction involving sex-role, gender schema, and Type A/B status was significant ($p < .05$) for females.

The college men failed to provide any sign of an interplay between the two sex-role variables, and, like the 1986 study of sex-role behavior, masculinity or femininity seemed unimportant in distinguishing between Type As and Bs. There was one effect in the male data that could be confirmed by statistical test ($p < .05$). Type A men, whatever their sex-role orientation, were less cognizant of traditional role expectations than Type Bs. Wherever male college students pick up the pattern of competitive, time-urgent striving for achievement, it does not appear to be from an overwhelming sense of what society traditionally expects of men.

The lack of agreement between the traditional and nontraditional that emerged when the social and gender-schematic aspects of sex-role were considered together for Type A women offers an interesting set of contradictions. What does it mean to find Type As made up of non-traditional masculine women sensitive to traditional sex-role stereotypes and traditional feminine women with minimal cognizance of society's traditional expectations? The paramount question is whether one or both of these paradoxical combinations adds to Type A vulnerability to cardiovascular disorder? The stress scores for the various sex-role groups, unreported in the original publication, allow me to examine risk. Table 8.9 includes the average stress scores of Type A/B females and males after a further refinement into the same masculine and feminine sex-role groups that gave us the unusual gender-schema results.

When the female results were examined, it was evident that Type As were under heavy stress whether they qualified as more masculine or feminine when compared to Type Bs ($p < .01$). College men produced the same Type A effect ($p < .05$), although excessive stress was noted only in the masculine Type A male. On the face of it, these results appear to be out of step with the conclusions drawn from the Heilbrun Palchanis, and Friedberg (1986) study into extended personality correlates of Type A status in college women. In that study masculinity was

Table 8.9.   Stress Reported by College Students Considered by Type A/Type B Status and Masculine/Feminine Sex-role Commitment

Sex-role Commitment	Females				Males			
	Type A		Type B		Type A		Type B	
	N	M	N	M	N	M	N	M
Masculine	12	58.50	8	38.11	10	50.40	12	33.08
Feminine	8	55.75	12	39.18	10	36.00	9	35.38

Note. - Unreported data taken from Heilbrun, A. B., Wydra, D., & Friedberg, L. (1989). Sex role correlates of stress-prone Type A behavior in college students. Sex Roles, 21, 433-448.

indicted as maladaptive and a presumed source of stress for female Type As as combining masculine instrumental qualities and Type A characteristics promised to compound competitive striving for success. However, the present results are more specific, since they direct our attention separately to the Type A women who have assumed a masculine identity and those who are feminine. When this is done it turns out that excessive stress can result from either adopted sex-role.

Finding gender-schema extremes for masculine and feminine Type A women in Table 8.8 and comparably high stress scores for these same groups in Table 8.9 suggests that the inconsistency between sex-role behavior and sensitivity to traditional role values is responsible for risk-conferring stress. However, the analysis most relevant to this conclusion has not as yet been reported. Table 8.10 presents stress levels for women and men, each gender broken down by Type A/B and then by the relationship between predominant sex-role behavior and strength of the gender schema (determined by median split). Relationships between these sex-role components were represented by three groups. Two inconsistent groups (masculine-strong gender schema, feminine-weak gender schema) included women whose untraditional sex-role behavior was out of line with their sensitivity to tradition or whose traditional sex-role behavior was coupled with a disregard for tradition. The third group of females included all who displayed better agreement between behavior and sensitivity to stereotype. The males in the sample were grouped in the same way.

Even though the breakdown of subjects resulted in uncomfortably small subgroups, statistics applied to the stress figures in Table 8.10 command attention. An interaction effect ($\underline{p} < .05$) emerged for college females. This can be explained by the very high stress levels for Type A women whose sex-role behaviors are inconsistent with their sensitivity to traditional roles of women and men. The same inconsistency is not related to stress when only Type B women are considered, nor was there any statistically-verified effect for men.

The conclusion regarding sex-role status as a specific risk factor for CHD, when associated with the Type A pattern in college women, is more complicated than I originally anticipated. No one (to my knowledge) has explored the possible intricacies of sex-role introduced by considering both behavior and gender schema concomitantly, and complication may be the destiny of those so inclined. My previous speculation had identified masculinity in Type A women as a risk factor, because its instrumental qualities reinforced the hard-driving, competi-

Table 8.10. Stress Reported by College Students Considered by Type A/B Status and Relationship Between Sex-role Behavior and Strength of Gender Schema

Relationship Between Sex-role and Gender Schema	Females				Males			
	Type A		Type B		Type A		Type B	
	N	M	N	M	N	M	N	M
Masculine-Strong Schema	6	63.00	6	35.33	4	42.00	9	33.11
Feminine-Weak Schema	6	61.67	5	38.80	6	34.67	3	44.33
Rest of Subjects	8	50.00	9	40.89	10	48.80	9	31.33

Note. - Unreported data taken from Heilbrun, A. B., Wydra, D., & Friedberg, L. (1989). Sex role correlates of stress-prone Type A behavior in college students. Sex Roles, 21, 433-448.

tive Type A pattern. The result promised to be an even more strenuous commitment to attaining personal goals, both short-term and long-term. However, since both masculine and feminine sex-roles that are out of synchrony with gender schema appear to be risk factors, my previous conclusion requires elaboration.

I continue to believe that the college woman who combines a masculine instrumental goal orientation with Type A competitiveness and time-urgency would place special priority upon goal attainment. Career success, the centerpiece of feminist gender-role revision, would assume an almost inevitable predominance in her hierarchy of goals. If the masculine, Type A woman is committed to revised roles for men and women, it would not be surprising to find that she is cognizant of traditional role assignments. Awareness of traditional roles is basic to informed revision for those who adhere to feminist doctrine. The relatively strong gender schemas displayed by masculine, Type A college females are not taken to mean that they are sensitive to traditional role expectations in the sense of conformance; just the opposite, their sensitivity has more to do with knowing what to avoid.

These same instrumental, Type A women would experience added pressure to succeed to the extent that they saw themselves as competing with men to validate the feminist view of equal (superior?) career potential. The absence of anything comparable to the role revision explicit in feminist doctrine or the gender rivalry that seems inherent in feminism could explain why the sex-role evidence for males was so bland. There is no obvious counterpart to sex-role/gender-schema inconsistency as a vital concern among college men as appears to be the case for women. Cognizance of the traditional male role is not a consuming passion for college men, at least for those who qualify as Type As. Recall that lower gender-schema scores were obtained for at-risk Type A men whether they were more masculine or feminine (see Table 8.8). Two studies now have told us that sex-role and Type A status do not interact with each other in college men whether we consider sex-role as a complex variable or not.

The feminine Type A college woman, who combines the expressive qualities of this sex-role with the aggressive competitiveness of the Type A, is a candidate for stress simply because these behavioral orientations are in conflict. You cannot extend warm feelings towards others and hope for reciprocity while at the same time harboring aggressive competitive inclinations at every turn. It stands to reason that a poorly-developed gender schema becomes involved in this stress-provoking pattern, since insensitivity to traditional role values would make it easier to adopt such contradictory tendencies. Someone out of touch with the ingredients of traditional role expectations might have an easier time taking on such an odd and dysfunctional combination as expressive warmth and aggressive hypercompetitiveness. The seeming problems in social relationships that were assumed for more masculine, Type A women when various harsh and alienating personality characteristics were identified may be matched in severity by feminine, Type A women. It is difficult for me to imagine what a feminine social style based upon expressive warmth and aggressive hypercompetitiveness would resemble, but many of the feminine attributes of Type A women included back in Table 8.5 suggest that the combination did not work very well -- "anxious," "faultfinding," "impulsive," "temperamental," "touchy," and "worrying."

Chapter 9

Type A Behavior, Stress and the Risk of Cardiovascular Disorders: Specific Risk Factors Related to Augmentation and Maintenance

This chapter will continue the consideration of studies in our Type A research program but will concentrate on evidence that seems especially relevant to other aspects of stress vulnerability and CHD risk. In Chapter 8 I emphasized the investigation of stress-arousing variables that most likely render their influence by increasing the frequency of competition for the Type A. Competition, in turn, was assumed to be intrinsically conducive to stress; the more frequently the person competes, the greater the arousal of stress. There was some lesser emphasis upon the maladaptive social qualities found as correlates of the Type A pattern in college women. Given their own harsh personality descriptions, it would be hard to imagine that the Type A female, especially the masculine version, would not suffer considerable arousal of interpersonal stress outside the competitive arena. Subsequent evidence isolated a subset of feminine Type As who gave evidence of their own brand of dysfunctional social transaction.

Perhaps a brief review of the arousal variables would be in order to help keep a growing list of Type A risk factors in mind. Three arousal factors were identified as contributors to hypercompetiveness. A deficit in self-control would create a problem in behavioral restraint no matter what the level of awareness might be regarding the folly of competitive excess. An external locus of control of reinforcement describes an attitude emphasizing the role of extrinsic factors in determining behavioral outcomes and minimizing the person's own sense of responsibility for reward and punishment. Applied to competitive situations, an external locus of control would lead the Type A woman to disregard her personal history of reinforcement in prior competition. Winning or losing, after all, is in her way of thinking largely a matter of luck, chance, fate, or the whims of those who establish outcome. Less governed by competitive history of wins and losses, the external Type A woman may lose the advantage of experience or even common sense in containing her competitive motivation.

Sex-role as the third risk-conferring arousal variable in Type A college women was a bit more complex, since it involved consideration of component variables that are rarely conceptualized together. In essence, what we found was that when sex-role identity was considered in terms of both behavior and sensitivity to traditional role expectations, masculinity and femininity each turned out to be a specific risk factor. In my judgment the finding that masculinity and sensitivity to tradition were paired in the Type A woman under greater stress derives from the independent contributions of a masculine instrumental orientation and Type A patterning to being competitive. Role sensitivity in the masculine Type A female reflects an awareness (and rejection) of the more passive stereotype for women; this negative standard serves to further motivate competitiveness. Feminine Type A females, on the other hand, were remarkably insensitive to role expectations, and the cultural proscriptions against aggressive competition would be ineffective. The stress that was noted for feminine Type A women would be generated not only by demonstrations of Type A competitiveness but also by their lack of preparedness for the cut-throat character of competition once it begins (an augmentation effect).

In this chapter I will turn my attention to variables that might increment risk by augmenting the level of stress usually associated with competitive situations or by sustaining stress over extended time periods to the point of chronicity. Before I do, I would like to remind the reader once again that the conceptual categories of stress arousal, augmentation, and maintenance are to some extent arbitrary, since some risk factors could contribute to Type A stress in more than one of these ways. The acid test of the risk introduced by a given factor remains whether it is associated with elevated stress in the Type A and not within Type B controls. Why the association occurs is a matter of interpretation and subject to eventual proof.

Risk Factors that Augment Level of Stress For Type As Within Stress-arousing Competitive Situations

It has been suggested that the burden of stress carried by Type As is not only proportional to the number of times that they are involved in stress-provoking competitional encounters, but also varies with the degree to which stress may routinely escalate within these situations. Everyday and long-range contests in which there will be winners and losers are abundant in the academic, social, and recreational life of the American college student. The search for factors governing augmentation of stress led us to consider what distinguishes between the Type A woman who can take these contests in stride and the Type A who cannot. Since all Type As are motivated to compete, why is it that some endure these win-or-lose situations with greater equanimity, whereas others seem unable to contain emotional distress?

Self-preoccupation as a possible stress-augmenting factor within stress-arousing competitive situations. Self-preoccupation has received prior definition as the tendency to interpret the world in terms of differences between oneself and others and to remain acutely aware of oneself while interacting with the environment. Preoccupation with self was found to be an important cognitive risk factor in anorectic development as well as menstrual dysfunction. This made sense in that both disorders involve the woman's special attentiveness to and concern for her own body or its functions. This aspect of self-preoccupation loomed as a specific risk factor for the female generally at-risk for anorexia, because it would allow an interest in body thinness and the effect of food upon her body to become an obsession. The risk introduced by self-preoccupation in college women experiencing some degree of premenstrual or menstrual distress seemed best explained in terms of excessive attention directed toward the menstrual cycle. This would lend itself to even greater sensitivity to this body system; increased sensitivity would likely add to the woman's discomfort and reduce her tolerance for menstrual changes.

A second basis for self-preoccupation seems to be required in order to make sense out of Type A risk, since bodily concern plays no obvious role in the dynamics picture for young-adults. Ego concerns, the priority accorded to self-esteem and to gaining the esteem of others, can certainly serve as an alternative source of self-preoccupation. Egoistic self-preoccupation would seem to be a paramount ingredient of the Type A's achievement-driven, competitive, time-urgent pattern. The self-preoccupied Type A woman should be even more attuned to her own goal-attainment and competitive outcomes than her less preoccupied Type A peer. With greater concern comes greater stress.

Given that preamble regarding the importance of self-preoccupation, you may find it disappointing that for the first and only time in this book on stress and disorder in women I will present evidence bearing upon a particular risk factor that was collected from an exclusively male sample. It is because I consider self-preoccupation to be such an important risk factor in stress-related disorder that I would rather depend on cross-gender generalization of results than ignore the implications of ego-investment for Type A risk in college women. It was an oversight not to have included college women when self-preoccupied Type As were studied in the first place. I am encouraged to make this departure from the usual exposition of Type A evidence, because the reasoning concerning self-preoccupation and stress in Type A risk is the same for women and men. Any Type A who is excessively ego-involved should be prey to surges in competitive stress and added concerns about goal-attainment.

Heilbrun and Friedberg (1987) considered the possible stress-augmenting role of self-preoccupation in Type As, using a sample of 53 males from the college population. The methodology of this study included the self-schema procedure detailed in the section of the book on anorectic risk. In brief, the laboratory task, presented in three parts over two days, measured the extent to which subjects remembered trait terms that they had identified as self-descriptive compared to trait terms that they deemed nondescriptive. The more vividly that personal characteristics are remembered, without regard to accuracy, the stronger the self-schema; the stronger the self-schema, the more the individual is sensitive to (preoccupied with) the self. Other measures were those standardly employed -- the stress-sensitive JAS Type A scale and the stress-symptom ratings.

Data analysis proceeded by dividing both the Type A and self-preoccupation scores at their sample medians, creating the four groups reported in Table 9.1. The average stress scores found in the table revealed the inevitable stress elevation for Type As ($p < .01$) but also a significant interaction ($p < .05$). The interaction resulted in large measure from the elevated stress reported by Type As who were highly self-preoccupied relative to other groups. They not only reported more stress than both Type B groups ($p < .01$) but more than the remaining Type As who were less self-preoccupied ($p < .05$). Type Bs with elevated self-preoccupation scores revealed the least stress among the

Table 9.1   Stress Reported by Type A and Type B College Males Varying in Strength of Self-preoccupation

	High Self-preoccupation		Low Self-preoccupation	
	$\underline{N}$	$\underline{M}$	$\underline{N}$	$\underline{M}$
Type A	16	49.06	14	38.36
Type B	10	30.00	13	36.15

Note. - Adapted from Heilbrun, A. B., & Friedberg, E. B. (1987). Type A behavior and stress in college males. *Journal of Personality Assessment*, 51, 555-564.

four groups; obviously, self-preoccupation is not generally conducive to stress.

These results emphasize the contribution of self-preoccupation to elevated stress but restrict this risk to competitive Type As. The implication is that once the self-preoccupied Type A becomes involved in the win-lose dynamics of competition his egoistic concerns begin to mount, outcome takes on even more significance, and stress escalates. It would be surprising if self-preoccupation did not contribute to the eagerness of the egoistic Type A for competing in the first place as new ways to validate self-esteem are sought. At least these are the conclusions to be drawn for male college students. I see no reason to conclude anything different for females.

Conflicting motives as a possible stress-augmenting factor within stress-arousing competitive situations. Sometimes in a program of research, as studies multiply, fortuitous discovery may play an important role in suggesting a new direction for investigation. This forthcoming series of studies, especially the first to be described, revealed many things to us for which we were not prepared by logic, theory, or the research of others. As it turned out, investigation into the motivation underlying Type A competitive behavior suggested a new reason why stress increases in the course of competition and yet another specific risk factor for the coronary-prone Type A.

The first study that considered the motives of Type A college students (Heilbrun, Friedberg, & Wydra, 1989) inquired into the various goals that might be important to the competitive Type A college student in the pursuit of accomplishment and recognition. It was anticipated that achievement motivation and the usual attainment goals in our society would assume paramount importance for the Type A. Our curiosity was directed primarily toward any secondary motives that might complement the achievement motive and be conducive to stressful competition. As it turned out, the achievement motive did not distinguish the Type A from the Type B but a conflicted pattern of secondary motives did.

The motivational analysis in the 1989 study began by specifying a number of goals that could serve as incentives in competition for the college student. A research approach was adopted in which the importance of these goals for CHD risk could be inferred from underlying Type A personality structure. In short, we looked for the presence of distinguishing personality traits in the stress-prone Type A that would promote behaviors geared to attaining one goal or another.

The rationale for specifying what motivates competition using personality traits actually involved two steps. The first step was to stipulate what goals may be satisfied through competition -- what competitors may be trying to accomplish by winning. We proposed five goals of competition, although it was not assumed that these necessarily exhausted the possibilities or that the motivational goals were mutually exclusive. Type As by competing may be striving for:

(1) <u>achievement</u> of success as defined by standard status symbols such as grades in school, salary or position in a career, rank in the military, or any socially-approved designation that denotes one person as superior in performance to others;

(2) <u>mastery</u> over others by outperforming them;

(3) <u>task proficiency</u> as when performing well in competition is reinforcing in its own right;

(4) <u>approval</u> from other people as a result of winning; and

(5) <u>aggressively outperforming others</u> so that they are made to look worse through losing.

The second step in specifying what motivates competition in personality terms was to identify personality traits that would predispose an individual to one or another of these five goals of competition. My choice of trait measures were the Need Scales for the Adjective Check List, originally developed by Heilbrun (1959) and subsequently included as a regular scoring procedure for the parent instrument (Gough & Heilbrun, 1965, 1980). These 15 scales were judgmentally derived using Murray's (1938) trait system, more specifically his list of traits for which the associated behaviors are most likely to be observable. The same manifest traits previously had been adopted for the Edwards Personal Preference Schedule (1957). Scores on the Need Scales are based upon the number of behavioral adjectives keyed as indicative of a given trait and selected by the subject as self-characteristic (plus items) as well as the number of items endorsed by the subjects that are keyed as inconsistent with the same trait (minus items). Raw scores (plus items less minus items) on each of the 15 scales are converted into standard scores with a mean of 50 ($\underline{SD} = 10$) by consulting college norms for females and independent norms for males.

Given the personality traits that were available from the Need Scales, the following scale patterns were proposed as critical to the five motivational goals for competition:

(1) Higher on the <u>Achievement</u> scale (predisposing women toward

achieving standard symbols of success and status);

(2) Higher on the <u>Dominance</u> scale (predisposing women toward mastery);

(3) Higher on the <u>Order</u> and <u>Endurance</u> scales and lower on the <u>Change</u> scale (performance-enhancing trait characteristics predisposing women toward task proficiency);

(4) Higher on the <u>Succorance</u> scale as evidence of greater emotional dependency (predisposing women toward gaining approval from others);

(5) Higher on the <u>Aggression</u> scale (predisposing women toward denigrating competitors by beating them).

The remaining eight Need Scales (see Table 9.2) were analyzed even though they were not directly relevant to the five proposed goals of competition.

Several simplifying steps were taken before the data were submitted to final analysis. The 81 subjects were defined as Type A or Type B based upon a median split of the sample distribution of 12-item JAS scale scores. The stress-symptom scores were divided at their respective mid-points for the Type As and Type Bs. Accordingly, stress-prone Type As in this study were put through two selection filters; they had to score higher on the special Type A scale, already shown to be related to stress, and also be higher on the stress score. A preliminary check for the 40 females and 41 males established that the results of Type A/Type B comparisons for women corresponded to those that were found for Type A men, so we combined results across gender. Finally, as the tabled data will show, low-stress Type As and both Type B groupings were quite similar in their personality scores. Accordingly, trait scores for these three groups, while presented individually for reader information, were introduced into a combined control group to simplify statistical comparison with stress-prone Type A subjects.

I shall try to present the results of our statistical analysis in as uncomplicated way as possible, since I know that Table 9.2 contains a cumbersome amount of information. First, let me narrow our focus by pointing out what was not found in way of Type A goals for competition. The absence of personality differences between stress-prone Type As and controls did not support the idea that stress-prone Type A students were distinctive in their achievement motivation (much to my surprise), that they competed in order to assert interpersonal mastery, or that they took special pride in how they performed on competitive tasks.

Table 9.2.   Mean Personality Scores for Stress-prone Type A College Students and Various Type A/B Control Groups

Personality Trait	Stress-prone Type As (1) (N = 22)	Low-Stress Type As (2) (N = 18)	Stress-prone Type Bs (3) (N = 21)	Low-Stress Type Bs (4) (N = 20)	Combined Controls (2-4) (N = 59)
Achievement	49.76	49.33	48.06	50.70	49.41
Dominance	54.32	51.06	50.06	54.15	51.84
Order	45.56	47.67	46.61	46.85	47.04
Endurance	46.20	49.44	48.11	48.25	48.59
Change	51.92	51.33	51.22	54.60	52.46
Succorance	51.60	49.28	46.83	44.95	45.88
Aggression	60.76	52.50	51.72	52.25	52.16
Deference	36.68	47.94	45.67	45.00	46.16
Autonomy	58.00	51.78	53.22	52.95	52.50
Nurturance	43.12	49.56	50.22	53.55	51.20
Affiliation	43.44	50.56	47.94	51.25	49.96
Intraception	44.48	50.05	52.39	52.90	51.82
Heterosexuality	54.68	56.28	59.06	60.15	58.55

Table 9.2 continued

Personality Trait	Stress-prone Type As (1) ($N = 22$)	Low-Stress Type As (2) ($N = 18$)	Stress-prone Type Bs (3) ($N = 21$)	Low-Stress Type Bs (4) ($N = 20$)	Combined Controls (2-4) ($N = 59$)
Abasement	44.80	47.78	46.00	43.05	45.52
Exhibition	58.80	54.28	51.39	54.30	53.36

Note. - Adapted from Heilbrun, A. B., Friedberg, L. & Wydra, D. (1989). Personality underlying motivation for Type A behavior in late adolescents. Journal of Youth and Adolescence, 18, 311-319.

The positive findings, on the other hand, included greater emotional dependency for the stress-prone Type As, as revealed by higher Succorance scores ($\underline{p} < .01$). The stress-prone Type A was depicted by this result as more reliant on others for emotional support, in line with the self-preoccupation of the Type A that has been discussed. Gaining emotional reassurance would feed an egoistic concern about being lovable, likable, or worthy of respect. The higher Aggression scores ($\underline{p} < .001$) that were found would be consistent with a denigrating quality to Type A competition in which the goal would be to psychologically damage the competition.

Just how compatible are these motivational findings with the prototype of the Type A woman (and man) inherited from the literature? As I have said, the finding that Type A women under the heaviest stress do not describe themselves as excessive in their achievement motivation came as a surprise. They were not less achievement-oriented than other college students, but neither did they display the burgeoning motivation to get ahead in life that was expected. On the other hand, the Aggression scale results came as no great surprise, since aggressiveness and the emotional accompaniment of hostility have been widely heralded as integral to the Type A pattern. If you consider what "aggressive" really means, not simply as synonymous with "assertive" but as seeking to inflict damage on a target, then aggressiveness within competition must include the intent to denigrate competitors. Returning to the unanticipated, there was no particular reason to expect greater emotional dependency upon others for approval, respect, and other supportive responses, at least from standard assumptions regarding the coronary-prone personality pattern. This finding might have been anticipated if egoistic self-preoccupation had been more carefully considered.

An intriguing possibility was suggested by the analysis of competitional goals in the Heilbrun, Friedberg, and Wydra study, and this is where serendipity prevailed. The combined presence of emotional dependency and aggressive goals would indicate a motivational conflict within competition for the stress-prone Type A woman if logic means anything. High aggression suggests that highly-stressed Type As enter competitive situations motivated not only to win, like most, but also to psychologically harm their competitors by beating them. High succorance suggests that competition may offer these same Type A women an opportunity to satisfy their need for approval, liking, and respect. It seemed to us that some degree of incompatibility exists between aggression and approval-seeking if the motives are directed toward the same people. Competing aggressively with the intent of not only winning but also demeaning the competition is not likely to generate the kind of approval, support, and warmth that the succorant woman would be seeking. If it could be shown that these motivational dynamics were actually represented in stress-prone Type A competitiveness, a conflict between aggressive and emotional-dependency needs could be assumed. Conflict in competition, in turn, would qualify as a stress-augmenting factor and as an additional specific risk factor for cardiovascular disorder. Follow-up research will be presented that explored these implications.

Although the remaining eight personality scales from the Adjective Check List were not part of the analysis of competitional goals, they did cast some light on the results already reported and on the more general social maladjustment that was inferred from the earlier (Heilbrun, Palchanis, & Friedberg, 1986; Heilbrun, Wydra, & Friedberg, 1989) analysis of Type A female personality. In regard to the results that I have just discussed, it is important to note that the emotional dependency (succorance) of stress-prone Type As flourished despite the fact that they were less dependent in the common sense of the term in which people look to others for decisions or guidance (instrumental dependency). Comparisons on both Autonomy and Deference scales confirmed the greater independence of coronary-prone Type As ($ps < .05$). This has some implications for the picture of social alienation that is building for at-risk Type As, but it also suggests that their emotional dependency occurs in subtle isolation from the Type As' characteristic independent social posture.

The remaining personality features that distinguished stress-prone Type As from the remainder of the college sample went beyond the hypercompetitive, striving, time-urgent prototype to include many dysfunctional traits that augured poorly for the general quality of their social transactions. As I observed on earlier pages, a problematic social life would add substantially to the stress that the Type A woman derives from her obsessive competitiveness and the new revelation of a possible conflict in competition once engaged. The analysis of the remaining personality variables provide corroborative evidence for the social maladjustment observed earlier in Type A women, although in the present study Type A males are implicated as well.

Stress-prone Type As in the present study showed themselves to be socially alienated based upon their personality profile, and they did so in every way possible within the limits of our analysis. They fell low on both <u>nurturance</u> (to give emotionally or materially to others) and <u>affiliation</u> (to engage in social relationships) relative to controls (p̱s < .001). I have noted the high <u>autonomy</u> and low <u>deference</u> (p̱s < .05) of the at-risk student that describe an independent person who will avoid reliance on others for guidance or material needs. All four of these trait findings reflect the presence of a masculine disposition (autonomy) or the absence of femininity (nurturance, affiliation, and deference). Low <u>intraception</u>, suggesting an insensitivity to the dynamics underlying behavior, bodes poorly for the interpersonal wisdom of the more at-risk Type A (p̱ < .05), and high <u>exhibitionism</u> (to seek the attention of others) reflects an unattractive substitute for mutual social transaction (p̱ < .05).

Given that we have had three sets of personality data portray the at-risk Type A female as socially dysfunctional above and beyond the problems of competition, a more compelling picture than for her male counterpart, some new observations seem warranted. If she attracts little reward from her social relationships, as I would expect, it follows that the stress-prone Type A woman would make an even more serious commitment to achieving career success through her hard-driving, time-urgent, competitive style. This helps to explain why she is so fixed in her ways; her striving for recognition is overdetermined. The seeming dysfunctional quality of her social life also puts the Type A's emotional dependency into clearer perspective, since she not only shares the career ambitions generally found in college women but also lacks social alternatives for diversion and attainment. The Type A woman at greatest risk nourishes a wish for approval, recognition, and liking despite the fact that she holds herself generally aloof from depending on others. This social alienation is likely predicated upon what the 1986 and 1989 studies portray as an abrasive interpersonal style (if she is masculine) or a dysfunctional combination of expressive concern for others and aggressive competitiveness (if she is feminine). Given such dismal prospects for satisfying her emotional dependency through normal social channels, the at-risk Type A female may have little choice but to seek satisfaction within the competitive arena. This kind of interpersonal opportunity may be all that is readily available to her.

Heilbrun and Mofield (1991) followed the 1989 motivational-analysis study by an investigation that focused more directly upon the proposed conflict in competition between aggression and emotional dependency for college Type As. It was important to reduce the gap between our assumptions based upon the research data and the behavioral reality outside of the laboratory that we were trying to understand. We chose to examine risk of stress-enhancement based upon conflict within competitive situations for Type A women from their own reported experiences in competition rather than depending upon the analysis of personality profiles.

A sample of 85 college women and 84 college men was collected by Heilbrun and Mofield, and the 12-item JAS Type A scale along with stress-symptom ratings were administered. A median split on the JAS scale scores distinguished Type As from Type Bs. A new procedure to get at competitional motives more directly was devised for the study. A self-rating questionnaire was used to recapitulate the experience of competition from the vantage point of the competitor.

The motivation questionnaire presented eight situations, familiar to the college student on campus, in which competition would be expected. The subject was asked to specify the importance of various possible goals for competing in each. These eight situations included competition:

(1) as part of a sports team,
(2) in a sports contest between individuals,
(3) in a classroom examination,
(4) for favor in a heterosexual relationship,
(5) in an election for student council,
(6) for a position as a dormitory counselor,
(7) for the lead in a student play,
(8) in seeking sorority/fraternity membership.

More specifically, subjects were told that the questionnaire would present several situations in which a college student would be competing with others and that we were interested in what their goals might be for trying to outperform rivals. The five motives for winning in competition that had been formulated for the initial study of traits underlying motivation, modified slightly, were used again. Clear definitions of mastery, task proficiency, need achievement, gaining social approval and respect, and denigrating rivals by beating them were provided. The reader will recognize the final two motives as translations of the succorance and aggression traits into the terminology of competition. It was predicted, based upon the preceding study, that these latter two motives would be more important in the competitive behavior of Type As who are vulnerable to high stress. There was no basis for expecting the other three motives to play a special stress-augmenting role for the

Type A woman or man given the previous negative results.

Subjects were asked to consider each competitive situation and to rank the motives in order of importance. The eight sets of ranks were scored inversely by order of importance: Rank 1 = 5, rank 2 = 4, rank 3 = 3, rank 4 = 2, and rank 5 = 1. The overall importance of each motive was determined by summing these rank values over the eight situations, so that a motive score could vary from 8 (least important in every case) to 40 (most important in every case). Each of the five summed motive scores demonstrated considerable variation across the sample. This suggests that they offered reasonable alternatives to the subjects in considering why they compete -- more attractive to some and less attractive to others -- since none was discarded as irrelevant by being ranked as consistently unimportant.

The seeking-approval and aggressive motive scores were introduced into a combined multiplicative index in order to ascertain how they vary in combination. To evaluate these two motives in terms of conflict, they must be examined in terms of how they function in concert. Conflict in competition would be suggested by elevations in strength of both approval-seeking and aggression motives within the same individual; a multiplicative index score would be sensitive to these individualized patterns. The distribution of motive-rating scores for approval-seeking, and independently for aggression, were transformed for the entire sample into standard-score distributions with a mean of 50 ($\underline{SD}$ = 10). The two scores were then multiplied. This transformation ensured that each component of the conflict index would have the same priority in determining the multiplicative score. Higher scores indicate greater conflict. For examples, a high approval-seeking score of 60 and a high aggression score of 60 would provide a very high conflict score of 3600; scores of 40 on each motive produces a very low conflict score of 1600.

Table 9.3 includes the stress scores for Type A and Type B women, broken down further by higher and lower scores on the conflict index using sample median-split procedures. The table also includes level of stress for Type As and Bs separated by mid-points on the three remaining motive scores. Type A females with higher conflict scores rated stress symptoms as more prevalent than Type A females with lesser motive-conflict index scores ($\underline{p}$ < .05). In contrast, no stress difference accompanied the split in conflict scores for Type B females. The prediction that motive conflict within competition would be associated with higher stress in the Type A woman was confirmed.

Table 9.3   Level of Stress Associated with Various Motives for Competition in Female Type A and B College Students

Motive for Competition	Type A				Type B			
	Higher on Motive		Lower on Motive		Higher on Motive		Lower on Motive	
	N	M	N	M	N	M	N	M
Seeking Approval X Aggression	17	50.12	29	40.04	23	37.40	16	36.75
Need Achievement	22	46.45	24	42.00	18	41.28	21	32.43
Task Proficiency	27	38.56	19	52.05	13	37.69	26	35.92
Mastery	25	45.00	21	43.10	15	32.27	24	39.17

Note. - Adapted from Heilbrun, A. B., & Mofield, K. (1991). Motives for competition in stress-prone Type As. Currently unpublished study.

Table 9.3 also makes it clear that achievement and mastery motives were not linked to level of stress within either the female Type A or Type B group; it actually came closer to this distinction within Type Bs. Task proficiency did show a reliable reversal of the stress results found for the motive-conflict score. It was the relative absence of a task-proficiency motive in the Type A woman that was associated with greater stress (p < .05). I will consider this significant result as soon as the evidence relevant to conflict in competition has been reported for college men.

The stress levels reported by Type A and B males, further sub-divided by median splits of sample motive distributions, are found in Table 9.4. The male findings provided a close approximation to what was found for the women in this sample. I could have combined the female and male data before presenting them, as I have done before under similar circumstances, but the replication of results was so striking that separate presentation seemed warranted.

Type A men who evidenced higher conflict scores reported more stress than their Type A counterparts who obtained lower conflict scores (p < .01); the conflict score had no relationship with stress level if the man was Type B. The prediction regarding conflict in competition and Type A stress held up for men as well as women in this sample. Achievement and mastery motives failed to distinguish the level of stress reported by either Type A or Type B males as was the case for females. Task proficiency provided the same reversal as was evident in the women's data. Type A men who were lower on the task-proficiency motive reported more stress (p < .05) than the remaining Type As, and no effect was noted for Type Bs.

The task-proficiency results, unanticipated but obtained for both the college women and men, suggested that Type As who lack the motivation to perform a competitive task well as an end in itself are those who carry the heavier burden of stress. The relative absence of artisanship, disallowing satisfaction from the quality of one's own performance without regard to contingent reward, considered together with an excess of approval-seeking point to an extrinsic goal orientation for the coronary-prone Type A. That is, goal attainment in competition is put largely in the hands of other people with less importance assigned to self-perceived quality of performance or self-approval. If this sounds familiar, it corresponds to what we found in separate studies of locus of control and self-control reported earlier. Type As with an external

Table 9.4.   Level of Stress Associated with Various Motives for Competition in Male Type A and Type B College Students

Motive for Competition	Type A				Type B			
	Higher on Motive		Lower on Motive		Higher on Motive		Lower on Motive	
	N	M	N	M	N	M	N	M
Seeking Approval X Aggression	20	55.10	21	38.14	23	31.30	20	37.70
Need Achievement	20	45.25	21	47.52	24	36.71	19	31.21
Task Proficiency	17	39.24	24	51.50	21	33.57	22	34.95
Mastery	22	47.68	19	44.95	16	35.19	27	33.74

Note. - Adapted from Heilbrun, A. B, & Mofield, K. (1991). Motives for competition in stress-prone Type As. Currently unpublished study.

LOC, who tended to view their reinforcements as controlled by outside forces, were more vulnerable to stress. Less effective self-reinforcement was found in the at-risk Type A as part of a more general deficit in self-control; Type As, then, were less capable of influencing their own behavior by self-generated reward or punishment. Now our findings suggest that stress-prone Type As view their reinforcements in competitive situations as tied to outside approval and not to self-reward. All three data sets suggest that Type As who looked away from themselves and toward others for their reinforcements are those reporting high stress.

If you reexamine the cell frequencies in Tables 9.3 and 9.4, it will be apparent that conflicted motives in competition are just as common in Type Bs as Type As, perhaps even more common. However, there is no indication of elevated stress in conflicted Type Bs, women or men. The term "conflict" in the case of Type B students qualifies as a misnomer; an "inconsistency without repercussion" seems more appropriate. In much the same vein, low task proficiency is amply represented in Type B women and men, yet it is not accompanied by high stress as was true when their Type A counterparts were examined. The evidence commonly requires me to consider why Type As provide the results that they do, but these Type B findings call for explanation as well.

In the case of the Type B, two factors are missing that contribute to high stress in the Type A with conflicted motives or low task proficiency. We seem to be considering a less profound dependence on extrinsic sources of reinforcement in the Type B, since emotional dependency, an external LOC, and limited self-reinforcement were found to be important only for the Type A. Then, too, we can be certain that the Type B is putting herself into competitive situations far less frequently than would be true of Type As. Whatever added stress may be generated within competition for the Type B who is conflicted in her motives or unresponsive to task proficiency is not going to have the same cumulative effect upon total life stress.

To summarize, the excessive reliance on outside reinforcement in competitive situations by aggressive Type As would inevitably expose them to these contradictory motives and to what I have designated as conflict. This Type A is hoping for approval and other emotional support from those she is trying to victimize by her aggressiveness. If the Type A is exposed to this conflict between approval-seeking and aggression within the competitive situation, I would expect stress to be augmented beyond that normally generated by contested goal-seeking. Considering the ubiquitous nature of stressful competition for at-risk Type A college students, it is little wonder that the added feature of conflicted motives generates high levels of daily stress.

Risk Factors that Maintain Level of Stress for Type As Over Time

The risk factors to be considered in this section of the book were subjected to study because of the rather obvious temporal difference in formulating vulnerability to cardiovascular disorder for the Type A college woman compared to anorectic or menstrual risk. A considerable amount of time must elapse before the modal 18-year-old we studied enters the age range when CHD problems become a more vital concern. At that early age anorexia nervosa is already a real possibility and clinical dysfunctions of the menstrual cycle a more imminent threat for those at-risk. Proposals regarding coronary risk for the Type A college woman must somehow bridge the span of time between her stress-promoting ways as a college student and the debilitating effects of stress upon the cardiovascular system that appear later in life. It seems likely that some of this discrepancy in time is illusory; CHD, at least when it results from too much stress for too long, may begin at a subclinical level well before the appearance of life-threatening symptoms.

There could have been an easier way to explain stress maintenance without invoking anything new about the Type A beyond the risk factors already covered. I could simply assume that the basic Type A personality pattern along with whatever cognitive or social variables we found related to higher stress levels in the Type A woman will remain as stable personality features as she moves through her adult years. Once a Type A, always a Type A, or something like that. I have no difficulty with this assumption, keeping in mind I am not discounting changes in risk-provoking personality traits for some women now considered Type As. However, I have to admit that the assumption of long-term behavioral continuity in the cases when Type A women retain their affinity to stress does have a convenient ring to it. Accordingly, it seemed worth our while to establish a more convincing risk picture by seeking additional factors that in themselves would serve to maintain stress over considerable periods of time.

As it turned out, the search for stress-maintaining cognitive functions resolved into an effort to identify mental operations that would influence problem-solving. We looked for cognitive traits that by their presence or absence would contribute to the continuation of problems that are responsible for the stressful life of the Type A college woman. To the extent that she is unable to resolve these problems or new ones that will arise in the future, stress will continue to be a familiar and potentially harmful commodity. The research already reported has made it clear that stress-prone Type A women are likely candidates for dysfunctions of ambition and social transaction. If it could be shown that the at-risk Type A lacked the psychological resources to be a capable problem-solver, we would be well on our way to explaining stress maintenance and discovering additional risk factors.

What are the types of personal problems that have come to light? I might start with the Type A pattern itself as posing a problem, but that may be too overgeneralized. Among the things that have been demonstrated in every study is that college women and men can adopt the Type A pattern without the stress that would signal a problem. However, if we concentrate upon only the stress-prone Type As, there is ample evidence of interpersonal quandaries that beg for resolution. Paramount here would be the seemingly insightless conflict in competition between the need to receive approval from those against whom the Type A is aggressively competing. Then, too, I could refer to the abrasive social traits endorsed by the stress-prone Type A woman that almost guarantee disruption in her social relationships. The specific problems may vary, but their basis in social alienation would be the same. The lack of synchrony between sex-role behavior and sensitivity to traditional values also could promote a variety of gender-role problems for the Type A woman under stress. Given the possibility of such wide-ranging problems, does the at-risk Type A woman lack the types of skills or the cognitive styles that could prove useful in recognizing, analyzing, and resolving these dilemmas?

Cognitive evasiveness as a limitation on problem-solving in stress-prone Type As. A person's ability to solve her own personal problems requires that a problem be faced, realistically appraised, and some plan of action devised that would alleviate the difficulty. My earlier discussion of coping styles that may be called into play when stress is aroused made the distinction between direct and indirect coping with the stressor. A direct strategy is usually better; by confronting the source of stress, it may be possible to bring about a change and neutralize its effects -- problem-solving at its best. Indirect coping styles do not address the stressor but rather act upon the emotions of stress and make them more tolerable. Some indirect styles are more beneficial than others. Exercise, for example, is a readily available way to reduce stress and promises physical benefits for the individual beyond controlling stress level. Alcohol or drug use may bring momentary relief from the emotions of stress, but the dangers of abuse and addiction with their impact upon life-style and health are serious hazards.

The psychological defenses are anotherderived by source of indirect coping readily available and much availed by the individual. Defensive styles allow the person to deal with the threat imposed by the symbolic representation of a stressor by distorting or otherwise avoiding its meaning. Our research (e.g., Heilbrun & Pepe, 1985) has found that the defenses also vary in their maladaptive effects judging by the level of stress accompanying characteristic use. Analysis of these defenses has led me to conclude that the maladaptive effect varies with the degree of evasiveness implicit in the particular defense. The more evasive the defense, the more likely it is that the source of stress will be ignored; the more a stressor is ignored, the less likely the person will try to cope directly with the stressor. Said another way, when you are faced with a resolvable source of stress, ignoring it is a very poor start toward solving the problem.

The most evasive defense that we studied was repression, the selective forgetting of distressing information. This defensive strategy allows someone to totally circumvent a source of stress, at least temporarily, by placing it beyond awareness. Repression as an evasive defense is bad enough, but matters can be made worse if other cognitive features that further limit access to sources of stress accompany its characteristic use. Repression would be more formidable and more conducive to stress maintenance when the person is unaware that she employs this means of distancing herself from troubling events by putting them out of mind. Selective forgetting puts a troubling thought one step away from awareness; not recognizing what you have done removes it even further from being accessible.

Conscious thought that is unreflective represents yet another cognitive characteristic that forms a barrier between problems and their resolution. Reflection, as I am using the term, involves the skill to think broadly about the relatedness of surface aspects of human problems as when the person considers how acting in fashion A leads to response B in another and eventual consequence C. Reflectiveness also involves thinking deeply about the underlying facets of a dilemma as when the person attempts to explain why A, B, or C would occur -- why people act as they do and why actions bring certain consequences. Both aspects of reflection should facilitate problem-solving.

Prior research has suggested a cognitive triad that is tied to excessive stress and, by my analysis, would be especially unconducive to addressing problems. The unreflective woman, given to narrow and superficial thinking, further protected from contemplation of problems by repression, with her defensiveness shielded by unawareness, should be especially vulnerable to poor problem-solving and the maintenance of stress. I would consider unreflective thought to be a deficit in cognitive skill, since I place special value upon this form of mental operation. Selective memory and lack of awareness regarding the use of repression appear best understood as cognitive styles -- the forms taken by our mental functions with no special value attached. Making the distinction between skill and style is academic, however, and has little bearing upon the issue at hand; do the cognitive qualities of at-risk Type As prepare them to deal with their stress-provoking problems?

Heilbrun and Renert (1986) examined the defensiveness of Type A college women in terms of their use of repression, low awareness of this defense, and unreflective thought. The laboratory procedures for measuring these three evasive cognitive qualities were described in the section on anorectic risk and will not be repeated here. We were interested in whether the Type A woman who possesses these problem-maintaining evasive qualities would be especially burdened with stress and at-risk for eventual CHD.

Heilbrun and Renert collected a sample of 68 college women (and 40 college men for comparison) and split them into the usual Type A/B groupings based upon median JAS scores. Preliminary analysis revealed that the pattern of relationships within each data set was the same for both sexes. This allowed us to combine over gender so that more stable groupings could be achieved.

Table 9.5 presents the stress means for Type As and Bs further subdivided by whether they scored higher or lower on the repression score using the sample mid-point on this laboratory task. An interaction effect ($p < .001$) within these tabled means was observed. Type A repressors reported the highest level of stress ($M = 53.83$), significantly more than Type As who failed to routinely use this defensive strategy ($M = 40.32$, $p < .001$). Type Bs demonstrated just the opposite effect; those who were more prone to use repression displayed less stress than Type B nonrepressors ($p < .05$). This reversal puts the evasiveness of the Type A in an especially clear light. It is the combination of using selective recall and having major problems to ignore that is associated with high stress. Side-stepping their problems, procrastinating at-risk

Table 9.5.   Stress-symptom Scores Reported by Type A and Type B College Students as a Function of Repression

Level of Repression	Type A		Type B	
	$\underline{N}$	$\underline{M}$	$\underline{N}$	$\underline{M}$
High	30	53.83	26	39.38
Low	25	40.32	27	47.85

Note. - Adapted from Heilbrun, A. B., & Renert, D. (1986). Type A behavior, cognitive defense, and stress. *Psychological Reports*, 58, 447-456.

Type As contribute to their continuation.

Table 9.6 takes our analysis of evasiveness one step further. The at-risk group of 30 Type A repressors was retained from the prior analysis, and the 78 remaining subjects in the sample served as controls. The at-risk group as well as the controls were broken down further by the sample mid-point on a score reflecting correspondence between rated everyday use of repression and actual use when observed in the laboratory. A similar breakdown of both groups was completed independently based upon reflectiveness. This arrangement of the subjects will allow us to determine whether unawareness of defense and unreflective thinking as additional forms of cognitive evasiveness add their own increments of stress for the at-risk Type A to that associated with repression alone.

The Table 9.6 data reveal that Type A repressors who are more self-deceptive about employing this defensive strategy reported singularly high stress ($\underline{M}$ = 56.50). This figure is well beyond that reported by Type A repressors more cognizant of using this defense ($\underline{M}$ = 42.72, $\underline{p}$ < .01). The same partitioning by repression awareness in the controls failed to bring about a difference. Lack of awareness added its own increment of stress to that associated with repression but only for the Type As.

Reflectiveness produced groupings of identical size as repression awareness and results that corresponded as well. Table 9.6 reports an interaction ($\underline{p}$ < .001) between group and level of reflection. Type A repressors who were also unreflective experienced greatest stress ($\underline{M}$ = 58.15), far more than Type A repressors who were more reflective in the way they processed information ($\underline{M}$ = 45.20, $\underline{p}$ < .01). The control group gave evidence of the opposite relationship as unreflective control subjects reported lower stress compared to their more reflective control counterparts ($\underline{p}$ < .05). Being unreflective seems to contribute to a calmer existence for the control college student; evasiveness seems to work in your favor if the problems you are ignoring are fewer and less compelling.

The general impact of evasive cognition upon stress level among Type As (and the clearest portrayal of risk for CHD) would best be determined within the Heilbrun and Renert data by splitting the total sample into those who combine all of the evasive cognitive qualities and comparing their stress-symptom scores with control groups. This also would provide a comparison between those who are most likely to procrastinate in resolving their problems and those who are less prone

Table 9.6.   Stress-symptom Scores Reported by Type A Repressors and Controls as a Function of Repression Awareness and Reflectiveness

Cognitive Trait	Type A Repressors		All Remaining Subjects	
	N	M	N	M
Repression Awareness				
Unaware	20	56.50	36	48.70
Aware	10	42.72	42	42.52
Reflectiveness				
Low	20	58.15	36	37.83
High	10	45.20	42	46.71

Note. - Adapted from Heilbrun, A. B., & Renert, D. (1986). Type A behavior, cognitive defense, and stress. Psychological Reports, 58, 447-456.

to do so. There were 13 subjects who were Type A and also were more repressive, unaware, and unreflective as defined by sample medians. These grossly-evasive Type As presented stress scores averaging 61.00. This is about as high as I have seen as a group mean on this stress instrument in my research into stress-related disorder within a college population. Average stress in excess of these numbers has been observed only when noncollege subjects bearing actual clinical diagnoses have been examined -- premenstrual syndrome in the case of women (Heilbrun & Renert, 1988) and post-traumatic stress disorder for men (Heilbrun & Handfinger, 1992). The remaining 17 Type A repressors, who in one way or the other did not demonstrate a full complement of evasive qualities, had a mean stress score of 48.35. The rest of the sample ($\underline{N}$ = 78), including the remaining Type As who failed to use repression and all Type Bs, evidenced a stress level of 42.62. The overall comparison of these stress scores revealed significant variation ($\underline{p}$ < .001). Specific statistical tests showed Type A subjects with the three evasive qualities to be more stressed than other Type A repressors ($\underline{p}$ < .05) and the larger residual group ($\underline{p}$ < .001).

In summary, this evidence suggests that when Type A women invoke cognitive strategies that allow them to minimize exposure to information of a disturbing nature, they are especially vulnerable to stress and at-risk for CHD. Evasiveness, whether it is accomplished by repression, diminished awareness of this defense, or a generally unreflective approach to information, would tend to compromise resolution of stress-provoking problems of any kind. You cannot solve problems or elements of problems as long as they remain beyond your awareness. Nurturing problems by ignoring them feeds into current stress for the Type A and promotes chronicity of her at-risk status. The evasiveness of control females suggested the opposite; the more evasive you are, the less stress you experience. If your problems are not profound, ignoring them seems to make life more tranquil. The findings for evasive cognition were the same for Type A and control men as would be the implications.

Social acuity as a limitation on problem-solving in stress-prone Type As. Evidence to this point suggests that stress-prone Type A women might falter in their problem-solving because evasiveness results in procrastination or insensitivity. However, this represents only one way out of many in which personality characteristics could interfere with solving personal dilemmas. Problems that are side-stepped by motivated forgetting come flooding back when relevant cues are confronted again; in most cases memories are set aside and not lost, as I use the term. Added to this, even generally unreflective Type As will consider the broader-ranging and deeper implications of their problems on occasion. When they do go beyond the obvious and superficial, they are likely to encounter bits and pieces that are crucial to understanding their dilemmas and resolving them. These are, after all, bright (by IQ test) college students that we have designated as stress-prone Type As. Before concluding such Type As are going to be so impaired in dealing with personal problems that they become vulnerable to chronic stress, we must go beyond the dimensions of evasiveness considered to this point. The next question is whether Type A women are also lacking in the cognitive skills that would help resolve social problems even when they do confront them? Social acuity, the term I shall use to include these skills, shall concern us at this point.

Earlier studies on social acuity in college students (e.g., Heilbrun, 1981b; 1982b; 1984b) will provide an important source of evidence for our current discussion even though the original investigations did not focus on the Type A personality. This realignment of earlier data is made possible by the later empirical development of Type A scales for the Adjective Check List by Heilbrun, Palchanis, and Friedberg (1986); this personality inventory had been part of the investigations in the early 1980s, although it was used with different measurement goals in mind. These derivative Type A scales for the Adjective Check List were not used in our Type A research program, because the JAS was available. Since they now will serve a valuable function as Type A measures, I shall briefly describe their psychometric properties.

The special JAS Type A scale was used to identify trait endorsements that distinguished stress-prone Type A from Type B college students with different sets established for females and males. The reader may recall that these differentiating terms were tabled in an earlier chapter as present and missing characteristics of the college Type A more likely experiencing heavy stress. These items were incorporated into separate scales with scores determined by the number of critical "present" items selected as self-characteristic added to the number of critical "missing" items that were not selected. The new Type A scales were found to correlate with stress about as well as the special JAS scale from which they were derived. It seems safe to say that the Type A scales for the Adjective Check List are workable substitutes for the JAS as a basis for selecting Type As who are especially vulnerable to stress (high scores) and their Type B controls (low scores). The availability of the derivative scales allows me to go back to the earlier social-acuity data and establish through reanalysis whether stress-prone Type As are flawed in their problem-solving skills.

Before reporting these reanalyses, I would like to begin the current discussion of social acuity by recalling one aspect of the personality trait data from the Heilbrun, Friedberg, and Wydra (1989) investigation of Type A motives in competition reported in the previous section. One personality comparison between Type As and Bs that was not central to the goals of competition received only brief comment but is relevant to any discussion of social acuity. The average Intraception scale scores for stress-prone Type A females and males ($\underline{M}$ = 44.48) and for a combined control group ($\underline{M}$ = 51.82) differed significantly ($\underline{p}$ < .001). This finding suggests that Type As vulnerable to stress make less of an effort to understand their own behavior or the behavior of others, the definition of intraception offered in the Adjective Check List manual (Gough & Heilbrun, 1980). Lower intraception in at-risk Type As would lead them to dwell upon what people do, the surface meaning of behavior, rather than the underlying dynamics of behavior including motivation.

A deficit in intraceptive behavior seems in line with what would be expected from stress-prone Type As who were found in another study to be unreflective people. While these cognitive variables were appraised by very different measurement procedures in independent college samples, both deficits agree in suggesting a narrowness and superficiality in the at-risk Type A's thinking. Lack of intraception (or reflection) would place a limitation upon the Type A's solution of personal problems to the extent that effective efforts at problem-solving depend upon considering the implications of behavior, especially motivation -- other people's as well as your own. Reticence to understand behavior should certainly be detrimental to the at-risk Type A woman beset by problems of excessive and conflicted competition and faltering social relationships.

Social insight is a second cognitive variable that contributes to social acuity. It has been defined as "the sensitivity to what others think and feel and the ability to diagnose or appraise the complexities or nuances of interpersonal relationships" (Gough, 1965, p. 155). This risk factor, more than any other I studied, seems to qualify as key to problem-solving in the social domain. Intraception, just discussed, represents the extent to which the person would interest herself in the intricacies of social behavior as a prelude to realistic understanding. When social insight is considered, such sensitivity is assumed as a shared property with intraception, but the person's skill in reaching accurate or wise decisions is also added to the mix. It is not difficult to imagine that a person could be heavily invested in gauging underlying behavioral dynamics or broad implications of behavior (viz., intraceptive) without being particularly insightful. The paranoid individual is a case in point. However, the opposite alignment -- social insight without an intraceptive style -- is unlikely. Social insightfulness is predicated upon skillful processing of many relevant details of behavior and situation and would not be expected in someone lacking intraception.

Social insight was measured by means of the Chapin Social Insight Test (Gough, 1965; 1968) in my earlier research. This questionnaire presents 25 social vignettes, and the subject's task is to pick the most appropriate, intelligent, or logical from among four weighted alternative solutions to these interpersonal dilemmas. Type A status will be defined by above-the-median scores on the independent female and the male Adjective Check List scales in this and the remaining social-acuity reanalyses. Table 9.7 includes the average social-insight scores for 55 Type A and Type B college women and for 34 male counterparts.

Two overall effects were noted in the statistical analysis of social-insight scores; women were generally higher in social insight than men ($p < .05$), and Type As fell short on insight when compared to Type Bs ($p < .05$). Of special interest, Type A women were less insightful than Type Bs ($p < .05$); whatever advantages college women generally enjoyed in social insight seems lost with the Type A. The same within-gender effect was found when the males were considered with Type As falling below Type Bs in social insight ($p < .05$). These findings for at-risk Type A women (and men) suggest a general impairment in processing social information and exercising critical social judgment.

In order to keep the emerging picture of Type A social acuity in focus, bear with a brief summary of our findings to this point. At-risk female Type As would be expected to deal with the obvious surface qualities of behavior and not with the complexities of underlying motivation or its broader implications (the intraception results). When required to appraise the complexities of interpersonal relationships, the stress-prone Type A woman should experience difficulties in reaching the right conclusion, since she lacks the skill for achieving insight into complicated social dynamics (the social-insight results). Either of these limitations would curtail the problem-solving ability of the vulnerable Type A female to the extent that understanding behavior and situations allows us to resolve problems. If understanding interpersonal behavior

Table 9.7.   Level of Social Insight for Female and Male Type A and Type B College Students

	Type A		Type B	
	N	M	N	M
Females	32	18.69	23	22.26
Males	17	16.18	17	20.18

is not important to problem resolution, then a lot of time in psychotherapy is being wasted. The results and implications for college men were the same.

Facial-decoding skill represents a third social-acuity variable available for reanalysis from my earlier research. Facial decoding allows me the identification of emotion being experienced by another person from cues available in the facial expression of that person. Skill in recognizing emotion would be important to avoiding or resolving personal problems in a number of ways. Being able to identify the emotions of other people would permit someone to respond more effectively to interpersonal situations, since it would allow the person to accommodate his or her behavior more appropriately to the emotional circumstances of an interpersonal encounter. Being able to read facially-expressed affect also would improve interpersonal sensitivity by offering clues regarding how one's behavior impacts upon other people. For example, an insensitivity based upon poor reading of emotional cues could contribute to the continuation of the Type A conflict within competition simply because Type A women and men do not appreciate how their aggressive efforts affect other people.

Facial decoding has been measured in several of my studies by means of slides portraying facial expressions of emotion posed by trained models (Ekman & Friesen, 1976). However, the data to be discussed here were obtained from an instrument derived by a slightly different set of principles, The Reading of Facial Expressions: A Self-test (Ekman, Friesen, & O'Sullivan, 1977). The multiple-choice Self-test was more promising for our purpose, because it was constructed to be more difficult and, therefore, more of a challenge to college students. College subjects find the slides to be quite simple to decode unless they are presented for unnaturally brief exposures. Facial expressions on the Self-test represent more complicated blends of two emotions rather than the single emotion found on each slide, and the subject has the opportunity to identify both. Blended emotional expression (e.g., anger and fear) is believed by test developers to be more typical of actual social transactions.

Table 9.8 reveals that Type A students, both female ($\underline{N}$ = 44) and male ($\underline{N}$ = 49), were less capable of recognizing emotions as registered in facial expressions on the Self-test than were Type B students ($\underline{p}$ < .05). Neither comparison considered separately by gender achieved significance. Again, the women were higher on this indicator

Table 9.8. Facial-decoding Skill for Female and Male Type A and Type B College Students

	Type A		Type B	
	N	M	N	M
Females	22	29.00	22	30.64
Males	20	24.80	29	27.53

of social acuity than men ($\underline{p} < .001$). Even though the Type A/B differences were not robust, we can detect a tendency for stress-prone Type As to be less capable of accurate facial decoding. This would imply that they will be missing or misrepresenting some important information that could help avoid or resolve social problems.

The final social-acuity variable that can be related to the Type A/B distinction using data from my research files is tolerance for ambiguity. This cognitive style reflects the degree to which an individual withholds the assignment of meaning to an unclear stimulus until greater clarity is achieved. Historically, low tolerance for ambiguity has received the greatest attention, since it was considered to be part of the authoritarian personality studied by Frenkel-Brunswick (1949; Adorno, Frenkel-Brunswick, Levinson, & Sanford, 1950). Early research made the case for poorer social competence in the person with low ambiguity tolerance. The inability or unwillingness to delay assignment of meaning in unclear social situations was thought to provoke premature conclusions, oversimplified views of the world, stereotypic thought, and an unwillingness to relinquish meanings already assigned. All of these point to superficial treatment of information in various guises. Superficiality could only detract from realistic understanding of people and their behavior and from the resolution of problems.

Although it has attracted less attention, the opposite end of the tolerance dimension also stands to detract from social understanding. Excessive tolerance of ambiguity suggests complacency or timidity when facing social uncertainties and signals a lack of motivation to come to grips with the uncertainties of interpersonal behavior. A high tolerance for ambiguity means that the person allows social unknowns to continue far longer than necessary, and deprives herself of information that might be vital to avoiding or resolving problems. As a cognitive trait, a very high tolerance for ambiguity would appear to be conceptually consistent with many other risk variables that have come to light in the analysis of problem-solving ability. High tolerance for the unknown would allow the Type A to elude potentially threatening social revelations in the same way repression, lack of reflection, low intraception, and missing or misreading facial cues provide means of escaping distress by failing to deal with social information. Social acuity and problem-solving ability suffer in each case.

The tolerance-for-ambiguity data I shall report was derived from a laboratory task (Heilbrun, 1972) based upon a procedure described earlier by Frederiksen (1966). The task was comprised of a series of 14 polysyllabic words that Frederiksen had chosen, because they attracted guesswork as to meaning when presented near auditory threshold (Blake & Vanderplas, 1950). A tape was developed for my 1972 study upon which each of these words was spoken in a normal voice nine consecutive times. The words were subsequently overlaid by masking noise with the noise reduced upon each repetition so that word meaning became progressively less ambiguous. The subject was told to guess the word when "reasonably sure" of its meaning. The tolerance-for-ambiguity score represented the number of times a subject withheld a guess prior to correct identification of a word, totaled over the 14 items. A very small score indicates an unwillingness to restrain guesswork until the words really become detectable and a low tolerance for ambiguity. A very large score suggests a willingness to delay interpretation of meaning well past the time necessary to be accurate.

Table 9.9 includes the tolerance-for-ambiguity scores for the 55 college females and the comparison group of 34 college males, each divided by median scores on the Type A scales. There was an overall effect for gender; females were more tolerant of ambiguity than males ($p < .05$). A within-gender effect was found only for the college women. Stress-prone Type As showed more tolerance of ambiguity than Type B controls ($p < .05$). Type A and B men showed low and almost identical scores. Stress-prone Type A women differ from all other groups, then, in that they have an unusually high level of ambiguity tolerance. This tendency to tolerate blurred meanings, to be satisfied with uncertainty, would impede ability to understand critical features of their social environment at any given point in time and would hinder problem-solving. Whether the failure to find Type A and Type B differences for the males would argue against tolerance for ambiguity as a risk variable is difficult to say. However, I would be prepared to argue that Type A men are especially penalized in their problem-solving by this general tendency for males to be intolerant of uncertainties and risk incorrect assignment of meaning because of their many other limitations in processing information. Being premature and wrong would be more devastating if it is not compensated by other problem-solving skills.

All in all, the intraception, social-insight, facial-decoding, and tolerance-for-ambiguity evidence culled from my files for reanalysis draws a consistent picture of flawed problem-solving for stress-prone Type A women. Type A men fared little better, perhaps no better at all. These limitations go well beyond repressive evasiveness and an

Table 9.9.   Tolerance of Ambiguity for Female and Male Type A and Type B College Students

	Type A		Type B	
	N	M	N	M
Males	17	39.35	17	39.53
Females	32	57.69	23	46.78

unreflective nature. Although at-risk Type A females protect themselves from confronting their stress-provoking problems by shunting
them aside when they can, these women will be limited in their ability
to solve problems even if they do confront them because they lack
social acuity. Analysis of social behavior tends to be superficial; social
insight into complicated interaction is lacking; vital interpersonal
information is lost, because facial cues communicating others' emotions
are not accurately recognized; and unclear social cues are too readily
tolerated. Lacking the social sensitivity that would make her adept at
interpersonal problem-solving, the female Type A seems destined to
keep old problems alive and initiate new ones. College men sharing a
Type A personality revealed much the same lack of social acuity in
addition to their evasiveness. Their prospects for problem-solving are
no better.

Competitiveness in Type A College Students and Stress -- an Integrative Study

As the final investigation of Type A risk was being planned, my
main priority was to add evidence regarding competition as a critical
feature of the Type A pattern. Several assumptions regarding how competition influences stress and CHD vulnerability for the Type A have
been necessary as I have attempted to place risk factors into an explanatory framework. These untested assumptions received attention in this
final integrative study.

Three questions were investigated. First, is competition actually
stressful for the Type A? This has been a paramount assumption in our
efforts to discover and explain new risk variables. It was based not
only on the presumed qualities of competition for most people but also
on the characteristics disclosed by research that would lead at-risk Type
As to augment level of stress in the course of competition. Second, if
competition proves stressful, does it make an appreciable contribution
to the daily stress burden of the Type A? Presuming competition to be
stressful for the Type A and to be a frequent event in her life has led to
the further assumption that it contributes significantly to a continuing
burden of stress and CHD risk. Finally, it has been assumed that the
motivational conflict within Type A competition is facilitated by
impaired social acuity. While it is tempting to conclude that
incongruous motives co-exist because of the limited social skills we
have found in the Type A, can this be demonstrated empirically?

Heilbrun and Karp (1992) conducted the final integrative study relating to Type A competition by administering eight psychological measures to a sample of 60 college women and 61 college men. Four of the measurement procedures concerned social acuity, and three of these were the same as used in the earlier studies that provided file data for reanalysis, reported in the previous section. The one exception was the measure of ambiguity tolerance where a psychometric scale was substituted for the time-consuming laboratory procedure to conserve subject time. This scale was developed by the criterion-group approach. The terms from the Adjective Check List that distinguished the self-descriptions of college subjects tolerant of ambiguity on the laboratory task from those provided by intolerant peers were identified using file data. These were combined into scales, separately by sex.

None of the correlations between the four social-acuity variables was particularly high over the entire sample. In fact, these correlations showed only about 4% common variance on the average; knowing how well the subjects fared on one social-acuity factor would allow you to predict only about 4% of the score differences on another factor. Accordingly, we were able to combine all four scores into a single social-acuity index without fear of redundancy. To do this, we transposed the four sets of raw scores into the same standard score distribution ($\underline{M} = 50$, $\underline{SD} = 10$) in order to give equal weight to each variable. High scores on this index of social acuity point to better problem-solving skills. For the women high scores reflected intraceptive qualities, superior social insight, better decoding of facial cues, and less tolerance of ambiguity. The male social-acuity index was constituted in the same way except greater tolerance of ambiguity was considered more socially acute and contributed to higher scores. This reversal in scoring seemed the best way to accommodate the gender difference on the tolerance variable found in the reanalysis of earlier evidence.

In addition to the metrics of social acuity, the Heilbrun and Karp study included the familiar 12-item JAS scale of Type A behavior and stress-symptom ratings along with a pair of rating scales constructed to get at the way that the individual experienced competition. These two scales involved ratings of stress from competition, examined from different time perspectives. One inquired into stress promoted by anticipating competition and the other required ratings of stress generated by competition itself. These were combined for purpose of analysis (after standard score transformations) into a single competitional-stress score.

The Heilbrun-Mofield (1991) technique for ranking the priority of goals in competition provided the eighth metric. Once we had a subject's rated priorities for the five goals, the set of ranks served as the basis for a motivational-conflict score. A conflict between motives occurs when both drives are powerful, and they are about equal in strength. Accordingly, motivational conflict in competition would be greatest when the rated importance of both emotional-dependency and aggression motives was relatively high and these ratings were close in value. The arithmetic procedure for deriving the conflict score took both requisites into consideration. The procedure involved adding the rated importance of the two critical motives among the five listed (i.e., rank 1 =5, rank 2 =4, etc.) and subtracting from this sum the difference in the two ranks. The first term represents the common strength of the two motives, and the second term represents their proximity in strenth. The highest conflict score of 8 would result from ranks of 1 and 2 for the critical motives with the final score given by adding 5 and 4 and subtracting their difference of 1. The lowest conflict score would be 2 resulting from one of the critical goals being ranked as most important and the other as least important $(5 + 1 - 4 = 2)$ or both critical goals being assigned the lowest possible priority $(2 + 1 - 1 = 2)$.

<u>Is competition stressful for the Type A woman?</u> The first analysis to be reported from the Heilbrun and Karp study has to do with the assumption that competition is associated with special stress for the Type A female based upon its intrinsic properties and her tendency to magnify stress in the course of competing. This assumption was tested by comparing the Type A women (above the JAS mid-point) with their Type B controls on the combined competitional-stress ratings. A comparable analysis for Type A and Type B males followed. Table 9.10 reports the stress from anticipated competition added to stress from competition itself. Female Type As experienced more stress associated with competition than did female Type Bs ($\underline{p} < .01$); the same effect was confirmed for males ($\underline{p} < .05$). Competition as a type of interpersonal encounter is a source of stress, at least if you are a Type A. Repeated frequently by demand of personality, it would provide a breeding ground for a burgeoning stress load in the pattern A college student.

<u>Does stress from competition make a significant contribution to daily stress level for the Type A woman?</u> A second analysis was required to strengthen the assumption that competitive stress in the Type A, just confirmed, makes an important contribution to general stress level in Type A women who are most at-risk for CHD. Female

Table 9.10.   Stress from Competition Reported by Type A and Type B College Women and Men

	Type A		Type B	
	$\underline{N}$	$\underline{M}$	$\underline{N}$	$\underline{M}$
Females	28	112.21	32	100.69
Males	35	111.06	26	104.31

Note. - Adapted from Heilbrun, A. B., & Karp, J. (1992). Deficient problem-solving skills as an explanation of Type A motive conflict in competition. Currently unpublished study.

Type As, who find competition more distressing and by their nature are frequent competitors, should have a singularly high general stress level and be at higher CHD risk. Table 9.11 includes the average stress-symptom scores for female and male subjects after breaking them down by level of stress from competition. The same median score served as the dividing line between high and low competitional stress for both sexes.

As is evident from the tabled data, Type A women who admitted to higher stress from competition also reported singularly high overall stress compared to other female Type As ($p < .01$) or Type Bs whether they identified competition as more stressful or not ($ps < .001$). Reading the results in a more dynamic way, the greater stress from competition for Type A women seemingly feeds into a risk-provoking general stress burden. No effect was evident for Type B females; very low general stress scores were obtained whether or not competition was rated as distressing. The Type B results make it clear that simply because competition is stressful for the college woman, it does not automatically convert into heightened everyday stress. The ubiquitous quality of competition for Type As but not for Type Bs must make the difference.

When males were examined, a different pattern of results was found. More stress from competition did tie in with a higher overall level of stress ($p < .01$), but this was equally true for Type As and Type Bs. In other words, stress input from competition was not found to be part of CHD risk provocation unique to Type A men in this sample as it was for Type A women. This gender difference can be shown in another way within the same data. Sixty-four per cent of the Type A women reported greater stress from competition, whereas only 38% of female Type Bs did. This proportional difference is reliable ($p < .05$); Type A women who are more stressed by competition not only report a singularly high general stress level but a proportionally high number of female Type As experience this seeming infusion.

If you examine the male results on Table 9.11, it becomes obvious that Type A and B men are not only the same as far as showing a competitional-stress effect upon general stress level, but they are also quite similar in the proportion reporting greater stress from competition. This leads me to reiterate something I said earlier when we examined sex-role in the Type A. It seems quite possible that being competitive is so pervasive as a male trait that it loses its impact as a distinct risk factor for Type As. The excessive competitiveness of the Type A women, however, may have more malevalent qualities, because

Table 9.11.   General Stress Levels for Type A/B College Women and Men Reporting Greater and Lesser Stress from Competition

| | Type A | | | | Type B | | | |
| | Greater Stress from Competition | | Lesser Stress from Competition | | Greater Stress from Competition | | Lesser Stress from Competition | |
Gender	N	M	N	M	N	M	N	M
Females	18	64.56	10	53.83	12	39.67	20	38.40
Males	18	47.83	17	38.12	12	44.17	14	35.71

Note. - Adapted from Heilbrun, A. B., & Karp, J. (1992). Deficient problem-solving skills as an explanation of Type A motive conflict in competition. Currently unpublished study.

it departs more radically from traditional behavior for females. It is hard to say whether competitive stress for Type A women is generated more by some internalized discomfort with the behavior or by the way others respond to hypercompetitive females.

There is one other critical feature of the women's stress scores in Table 9.11. Even though the average daily stress of Type A females who reported less competitional stress was reliably less than the extreme presented by Type As more distressed by competition, it was still quite high in terms of absolute value ($\underline{M}$ = 53.83) and elevation relative to both Type B groups ($\underline{p}$s < .001). This finding should remind us that interpersonal discord has been identified as a source of stress for the at-risk Type A College woman above and beyond what would be generated by competition alone. Even when stress from competition is said to be low, the Type A woman depicted by Table 9.11 seems to experience considerable distress from her dysfunctional lifestyle. This stands in stark contrast with Type A males. They earlier revealed no disruptive social traits comparable to those found for their female counterpart, and in this study reported high daily stress only when stress from competition was in evidence.

Is motivational conflict within competition related to impaired social acuity for the Type A woman? The third analysis shifts away from the assumptions regarding stress from competition and its significance for general stress level to the motivational conflict between the Type A woman's need for approval and her aggressive goals in competition. It was assumed that a documented deficit in social acuity for females and males would not only contribute to the chronicity of stress as problems persist but also would help explain why the Type A was host to two such incompatible motives as emotional dependency and aggression.

The assumption that limited social acuity would be related to motivational conflict was tested by splitting the Type A and Type B women at the median motive-conflict score and examining the resulting four groups for degree of social acuity. The same treatment was extended to the male subjects. Before I present these results, I would like to report the relationships between motive-conflict scores and general stress symptoms for Type As and Bs in order to reconfirm the status of motivational conflict as a risk factor.

Table 9.12 offers some explanation for why the male results have been less than robust thus far in the Heilbrun and Karp study. Statistical analysis of the tabled data revealed a singular elevation in general

Table 9.12.　General Stress Levels for Type A/B College Women and Men Reporting Stronger and Weaker Motivational Conflict in Competition

Gender	Type A				Type B			
	Stronger Motive Conflict		Weaker Motive Conflict		Stronger Motive Conflict		Weaker Motive Conflict	
	N	M	N	M	N	M	N	M
Females	17	67.71	11	53.71	13	41.43	19	36.89
Males	16	43.12	19	43.11	15	41.00	11	37.73

Note. - Adapted from Heilbrun, A. B., & Karp, J. (1992). Deficient problem-solving skills as an explanation of Type A motive conflict in competition. Currently unpublished study.

stress for Type A women who experience stronger conflicting motives in competition ($\underline{M}$ = 67.71); their general stress level was higher than other Type As with weaker conflict ($\underline{p}$ < .001) or Type Bs with stronger or weaker conflict ($\underline{ps}$ < .001). The apparent input of stress from conflicted competition into daily stress level is observed only in Type A women, since nothing emerged from the analysis of male data. Motive conflict did not qualify as a source of stress for Type A men. In fact, being Type A was not even associated in a statistical sense with elevated stress for men in this particular analysis, although it was in the analysis of data from the same males reported in Table 9.11. These may have been fluke sampling fluctuations, but they are consistent with my view that Type A risk dynamics may have achieved a sharper focus in recent years for college women than is the case for men.

The final analysis brings us to the heart of the issue regarding conflicted motivation in competition. Can a deficit in social acuity be found that would explain why the Type A woman would entertain two such conflicting motives in competition as emotional dependency and aggression? Type A and B women, again split by level of motive conflict, provided the social-acuity scores included in Table 9.13. The social-acuity averages for the four male groups are presented as well.

Type A women whose ratings suggested stronger conflict of motives within competition demonstrated a singular deficit in social acuity when compared to Type A women without such conflict ($\underline{p}$ < .01) and to Type B women who did or did not appear to be motivationally conflicted ($\underline{p}$ < .01). Looked at another way, the female Type A with stronger conflict was uniquely penalized by poorer social acuity that would deter her from identifying the nature of her conflict in competition or, if identified, would limit the problem-solving ability that could be brought to bear in resolving the conflict. No such difference in social acuity was found in Type B women who were more and less conflicted.

Exactly the same conclusions can be derived from the analysis of male data in Table 9.13 except the statistical differences were less robust ($\underline{ps}$ < .05). Oddly enough, male Type As realigned themselves with their female counterparts as far as explanation of motive conflict was concerned. Type A men who reported conflicted motives within competition revealed the same unique deficit in social acuity relative to their peers as did the female Type As. Why Type A college men come to harbor incompatible motives can be explained by their limited social acumen. Why this incongruous pair of motives was not associated with

Table 9.13.   Problem-solving Skills[a] in Type A and Type B Females and Males as a Further Function of Motivational Conflict in Competition

	Type A				Type B			
	Stronger Motive Conflict		Weaker Motive Conflict		Stronger Motive Conflict		Weaker Motive Conflict	
Gender	N	M	N	M	N	M	N	M
Females	17	187.94	11	209.09	13	208.92	19	210.79
Males	16	189.69	19	206.11	15	202.60	11	196.00

[a]Composite score based upon intraception, social insight, facial decoding, and tolerance of ambiguity as social-acuity factors.

Note. - Adapted from Heilbrun, A. B., & Karp, J. (1992). Deficient problem-solving skills as an explanation of Type A motive conflict in competition. Currently unpublished study.

extraordinary stress for these men remains unanswered except to note (again) that the interpersonal aspects of a Type A lifestyle do not seem as important for males as for females.

Overview of the Heilbrun and Karp results. The four analyses of the Heilbrun and Karp evidence lend support to the importance of competition as a source of stress and CHD vulnerability for the at-risk Type A college woman. They also offered empirical support to a number of assumptions that are important to the understanding of Type A risk from my perspective. These analyses tell us: (1) Competition is especially stressful for the Type A woman; (2) stress from competition seems to feed significantly into her general stress level; (3) motivational conflict between emotional dependency and aggression within competition is critical for the Type A female as far as incrementing general stress level and promoting CHD risk are concerned; and (4) lower social acuity is present in the Type A reporting motive conflict and could account for less ability or willingness to identify or understand her irreconcilable goals in competition.

The case for Type A males based upon the same kind of analyses is a more uncertain one. Male Type As reported more stress from competition than Type Bs. However, when those experiencing more and less competitional stress were compared on general stress level, both Type As and Type Bs more stressed by competition also were more generally stressed. Stronger motive conflict in competition was not associated with greater stress in general for Type A males, although this conflict was linked to a deficit in social acuity. While I am not tempted to relinquish interest in Type A risk for the college male in light of the considerable amount of positive evidence disclosed in our program of research, it is the female Type A college student whose dynamics stand out in bolder relief as provoking risk for stress-related CHD.

Chapter 10

Stress and Female Risk of
Psychobiological Disorder

With the discussion of conceptual framework, research methodology, programmatic data, and statistical analysis behind us, this chapter offers me a final opportunity to reflect upon what has been accomplished by the stress-and-disorder research and what has not. Our purpose, when we began exploring predisposition to disorder in college women under stress, was to identify specific behavioral attributes that could serve as early-warning signs. These risk factors might then allow for prediction of a future disorder coupling emotional anguish and bodily dysfunction. Having been involved with college mental health services and research for about 30 years before the stress-and-disorder investigations were initiated, I already was convinced that some college women were exposed to tremendous achievement pressures. Furthermore, I viewed the situation as becoming more acute by the 1980s as the mandate of individual attainment heralded by the women's movement became institutionalized. It followed that college women would be vulnerable to the effects of excessive stress. The challenge was to develop a research strategy that would allow us to discover which features of personality might identify those who run the risk of one disorder or another because of exposure to stress.

It is this research strategy that I shall turn to first. Although it was given considerable attention at the beginning of the book, readers now have had the opportunity to judge for themselves the quantity and quality of evidence that has been generated by applying the at-risk method. It seems to me that the credibility assigned to this research approach could fall at three levels. The nihilistic view would be that the research procedures used in studies of normal college women and assuming disorder before the fact can generate nothing that is meaningful or reliable; thus, any claim to prediction and improved understanding of disorder is automatically forfeited. Such an extreme view seems to pale in the face of the ponderous number of significant results that came to light in the course of our investigations. Even more compelling, these risk factors made sense as far as the dynamics and symptom picture for specific stress disorders were concerned. A challenging question for anyone inclined to this view is why the harvest of results was so bountiful and what their aggregate meaning might be if the data have no relationship to stress and disorder?

An intermediate view of the at-risk strategy might be that it is capable of revealing a great deal about the personality basis for current stress, but whether it can establish risk for future disorder is in doubt. While this is not my opinion, it does present an interesting and constructive alternative to my conclusion that our studies provide a basis for anticipating disordered psychobiological conditions in women. Even if it were true that we have not identified risk factors for stress-related disorders, the fact that our research provides a more complete picture of stress effects among young-adult college women represents progress. Stress is not only a harbinger of future serious disorder, but it also is a source of discomfort and anguish in the here and now. Revealing personality correlates of current stress in college women is a step taken toward improved coping with this maladaptive product of ambition, competition, and uncertainty in young women.

The third view of the at-risk research method would allow for the possibility that these personality correlates of stress can serve as early-warning signs of future stress-related disorder and have prognostic value as risk factors. There are compelling reasons to endorse this view. One is the parallel between the at-risk methodology and the "high-risk" research method that has gained considerable status as a way of studying premorbid development in schizophrenia. In high-risk research, the children of one or two schizophrenic parents are studied well before this disorder usually makes an appearance. Genetic studies have confirmed that the premorbid sample of children will contain a higher percentage of those who will eventually become schizophrenic than would a sample selected at random from the general population. Higher risk would make expensive longitudinal investigation of premorbid development a more feasible research investment.

The at-risk method, like its high-risk predecessor, also attempts to create a sample of subjects who will be at higher risk for a given disorder than would be true for a random sample from the same population. Instead of utilizing family history as the marker of vulnerability, however, the at-risk procedure depends upon the presence of behavioral attributes that would be expected during the subclinical prelude to a specific stress-related disorder. These have included the budding behavioral properties of the disorder itself along with high levels of stress. After this critical at-risk group has been identified, correlated personality factors can be sought by comparisons with appropriate control groups. Most commonly, facets of personality were investigated as risk factors by pairing them with preclinical behavioral properties of the disorder and using elevations in stress as a barometer of additional risk. These personality risk factors, largely cognitive in nature, were not chosen haphazardly. They qualified as reasonable possibilities in the search for behaviors that might increase the risk of stress-related disorder. Reasonable to me meant that behavior provided a fit to the known symptoms of each disorder or offered a logical basis for symptom development.

It is evident that the at-risk method for exploring vulnerability factors in a given disorder transforms at some point into a theoretical model for explaining the causes of that disorder. Start with a full description of the personality factors that introduce risk, as defined by increments of stress in women who show the seeds of disordered behavior. Complement this delineation of factors by specifying their relationships with each other and their combined effects upon stress. Place both the array of factors and their interactions into a broader socio-cultural context that elaborates the meaning of the personality configuration. Accomplish these things and you will have a personality theory of stress-related disorder.

The exposition of evidence in this book has progressed only so far in meeting the requirements for claiming theoretical status. Certainly, many specific risk factors remain unspecified, only a few of the higher-order relationships between specific factors have been explored, and the proposed socio-cultural context regarding competitive achievement-striving in our country was not subjected to investigation. A conservative view of the evidence seemed in order; taken literally, the discoveries are offered as empirically-based indicators of risk for stress-related disorders in college women rather than explanations. However, the fact that the risk variables could be readily explained as contributors to each disorder placed the findings beyond "dust-bowl empiricism." That they provided reasonable explanations for symptom development should at least lend added credibility to the risk factors that were uncovered even if a developmental theory of disorder is not presumed.

To be conservative at this stage of disclosure regarding the evidence from our studies is not to be taken as a bailout. I believe the findings to date are important and that their implications deserve attention, but I have a preconceived idea about the most likely audience for this book. I have not geared my writing, especially the presentation of studies, to the academic scholar/scientist. If I had, there would be a far greater emphasis upon methodology, statistical options, problems of inference, conflicting or converging evidence in the literature, and, of course, a more extended advocacy of personality and cultural assumptions. My hope for the scholar/researcher audience is that there is enough of substance in the book to stimulate theoretical interest and spark further research.

However, this book has been written for a different consumer. I have looked toward those who share a professional interest in the psychological well-being of college women in particular as well as other adolescent or young-adult females who contend with the stress of competing for critical social and career goals. Hopefully, these professionals will find the delineation of risk factors for anorexia nervosa, disorders of the menstrual cycle, and Type A-based cardiovascular problems to be helpful in individual cases where stress appears to be an important feature of the behavioral picture. These factors, to the extent they involve modifiable behaviors, offer a basis for amelioration of stress and early intervention in the progression toward serious disorder and bodily dysfunction.

Prior to discussing the differences in stress-personality interaction that distinguish risk for the three stress-related disorders in women that were studied, I will restate the socio-cultural context and underlying premise that I believe to be common to the various patterns of vulnerability. Before there can be stress-related disorder, there must be stress at a level capable of activating behaviors that could eventually prove psychobiologically disabling if left unchecked. I focused my research efforts upon young-adult college females, most of them 18-year-olds, as a generally stress-prone population. Part of this assumption was based upon commonplace campus observation that these women (along with their male peers) are exposed to the pressures of ambition and striving for success through competition. Most are now in college as evidence of their motivation and as an investment in their future as adults. The time has come to satisfy their own expectations and those held by family and friends.

This is not the whole story for the contemporary female, however. Many experience added pressure generated by the increased career opportunities for women. Women not only want to be successful,they are free to pursue professional success with far fewer constraints than before the 1970s. Unavailable opportunity no longer serves as a rationalization for not striving to succeed. To make matters worse for themselves, however, some women feel they must surpass men to be successful or to demonstrate female superiority.

If the added pressure for career success facing current college women were not enough, its requirements and uncertainties may be especially stressful for another reason. As female career opportunities have increased, so has the perception that a full commitment to achieve that goal may come at the cost of marriage and family, at least the quality of marriage to which they aspire. This conflict may or may not turn out to be realistic in the individual case, but that is beside the point. These are mostly 18-year-olds who were studied, and their current concerns hinge upon uncertain outcomes that lie years ahead. Since considerable priority is assigned to both social achievement and career attainment as future goals by college women, the conflict can increment stress for those who sense this impasse whether the perception turns out to be realistic or not. Men have no basis for anticipating conflict between career and marriage, and in fact, may believe just the opposite -- that their marriage of preference and successful family involvement depend upon career success.

Stress Dynamics and Stress-Personality Interaction in Anorectic Risk

Stress has been conceptualized as an aversive state involving two components. A cognitive component allows an awareness of threat and, more often than not, includes a specification of its source. An emotional component is triggered automatically by the threat and is responsible for the discomforting feelings that give stress its unpleasant character. I have assigned the emotional component of stress a major role in generating risk for a future lapse into disorder. However, I have proposed distinct ways in which stress can serve a pathogenic end; each type of stress dynamic contributes a somewhat different risk picture. If stress acts differently in the way it contributes to risk for varying disorders, the implications for intervention in the progression toward disorder would be expected to vary.

Stress dynamics. In the case of anorectic risk, stress is viewed as important to the extent it motivates behaviors aimed at escaping its emotional tension. Humans are basically hedonistic in that they usually will seek to avoid the arousal of unpleasant emotional responses. Since it is impossible to accomplish this completely, most of us settle for ridding ourselves of unpleasant emotions once they arise or at least reducing their aversive impact. The emotions of stress, then, are responsible for a variety of behaviors that have the reduction of emotional tension as a primary goal. These coping behaviors are conveniently broken down into direct and indirect depending upon whether they address the source of stress or simply represent ways of temporarily alleviating the aversive emotions.

The tension-reduction basis for anorectic development has been presented as part of a direct coping effort gone wrong. The at-risk college woman is faced with stress that is fostered by her perceived lack of progress toward standard goals of achievement, as this progress is gauged through her perfectionistic eyes. The at-risk woman's solution is to relinquish these goals and substitute something more attainable -- a thin body -- as she strives to lighten her burden of stress. The transitional stage involving an exchange of primary goal commitments would qualify logically as a period of mounting anorectic risk. During this period the woman weighs the merits of goal substitution at some level of awareness, and various cognitive and social risk factors are given the opportunity to enhance food restraint and make diminished body size a reality.

Unfortunately for the vulnerable female, the substitution of goals is unlikely to provide relief from the stress that motivated it. A sense of failed accomplishment is unlikely to be totally dismissed, especially if she remains in an achievement-oriented environment like college. In addition, concern regarding food and weight-loss assumes priority, and a new source of stress is generated. Continued stress following goal substitution opens the way for a tension-reduction agenda in which instrumental elements of body-thinning serve to increase and relieve tension. Eating precautions and restraint serve to relieve stress just as eating temptations and lapses promote it. Weight loss and an angular body image will also be tension-reducing as they signal progress toward the substitute goal. Ironically, the personality factors that begin to play a prominent role in the woman's pursuit of a thin body may have a perverse effect upon stress. Body distortion, for example, serves as an important source of motivation in food restraint and should contribute to achieving the goal of actual body thinness. However, rather than serving a constructive purpose for the at-risk woman and allowing her to relieve her burden of distress, this misperception promotes concern and stress within the dynamics of a stress-related disorder.

Intervention into anorectic risk, in light of the stress dynamics that I have sketched, could assume either (or both) of two directions. The diminished status of standard achievement goals has resulted in important measure from a self-deceptive perfectionism that casts a pall over career-related preparations. The fact that career progress falls short of perfectionistic standards is accompanied by a distrust of interpersonal relationships. Both lend pessimism to the woman's career and social projections into the future and make it no mystery why she is reticent to assume adult roles. In short, stress from the sense of failed accomplishment and dim hopes for the future is partially based upon distortion and should be subject to more realistic appraisal by the at-risk female.

Once distorted perceptions are modified and stress is reduced to a more tolerable level, there ought to be less motivation to pursue a new and trivial form of achievement that poses danger for the at-risk woman. If the perfectionism and distrust are derived from the unrealistic standards of others who continue to exert their influence over the college woman, most likely the parents, modification becomes that much more complicated. Adding further to the formidable challenge of what would be a reality-based intervention is the fact that the troubled woman is not simply harboring a focused and transient distortion of perception that requires therapeutic attention. Given the developing behaviors that place her at anorectic risk, it is clear that the vulnerable female is subject to misperception at every turn. She not only flaunts reality as far as achievement, social relationships, and body size are concerned, but her internal sensations are subject to gross distortions as well. Misperception in the college woman at anorectic risk is an entrenched and far-ranging psychological flaw.

Given that a shift in goals already has occurred and eating constraint prevails as a central focus, stress is generated by the concerns of attaining the goal of body thinness. Stress under these circumstances is likely to serve as a source of motivation toward the eventual goal, just as it may serve to maintain achievement efforts for those who pursue any desired goal. Stress can energize the efforts of the female to achieve bodily thinness just as it contributes to the striving for educational goals, career achievement, and social accomplishment. Of equal importance as a facet of motivation and more readily overlooked, briefly-enjoyed reductions in stress can reinforce the instrumental acts that are required to progress toward the goal of a thin body. Any behavior, including thought processes, that promises weight loss or the avoidance of weight gain may be rewarded and strengthened by the temporary reduction in unpleasant emotions of stress. This is no different than would be true for instrumental acts within any goal-directed sequence as when study practices become more ingrained when a good grade reduces stress associated with school achievement.

There is an ominous note struck when considering how stress may play a tension-reducing motivational role in eating constraints for the at-risk female, however. It is not just the more obvious instrumental behaviors associated with weight loss that are reinforced by a temporary drop in stress -- making out eating plans, avoiding meals, buying the right foods, etc. Given the strong association between food and eating, each time food is not eaten when temptation impels her allows the resistance of the at-risk female to be rewarded and strengthened by a drop in stress aroused by the possible breach in her restraint. Said more simply, every time she even entertains the thought of ingesting food, putting the thought aside may serve as a reward. These temporary but frequent reductions in stress made possible by avoidance of eating or even putting aside the thought of food would provide a system of self-generated reinforcement within the anorectic progression that strengthens dietary restraint. In principle, this accessibility of momentary reward through stress reduction would only be available because of the critical importance of a thin body to the woman at-risk for anorexia. Stress must be readily generated by cues associated with food to be available for frequent temporary reductions.

Disrupting this motivational pattern brought about by surges of elevated stress and its momentary relief, using whatever means available to the intervening professional, should prove beneficial, since stress is serving a dual motivational role and overdetermining food restraint. It is driving the woman toward achieving thinness as a goal by its presence and rewarding acts of food restraint by its absence, if my analysis is correct. It could prove difficult to implement that kind of intervention, given the difficulties in modifying the nuances of motivational dynamics with techniques currently available. Perhaps behavior-modification procedures could be applied, since the underlying cognitive/emotional constituents of the problem may be beyond volitional control for the college woman bordering on a full-blown anorectic disorder.

Difficulties in effecting change in this motivational pattern might be expected for another reason. The at-risk female may be reluctant to relinquish even a dysfunctional drive toward thinness or the reinforcement gained from weight loss or food restraint, since her previous experience has offered nothing comparable in way of goal attainment or available reward within standard domains of achievement. This to me is the essence of the common clinical observation concerning the importance of gaining control by the anorectic. She now controls her own goal attainment and reinforcements, as dysfunctional as they may be, and is no longer dependent on what might or might not be available from extrinsic sources. Her penchant for misperception (i.e., poor reality-testing) may even prevent her from recognizing the dysfunctional qualities of her motivation and make the trade-off even more attractive.

Stress-personality interaction. The contribution of personality to the risk of anorexia nervosa came into clear focus as the research program progressed. The pattern of risk variables was compelling not only because it was rather voluminous, based upon empirical evidence from many independent studies, but also because the risk pattern represents an entirely logical explanation of anorectic vulnerability. It was this simple. College women who were at greatest risk for anorexia were those whose personality traits would make it more likely that they would experience achievement problems and fail to resolve them, that they would fall back on body thinness as a substitute goal, and that their efforts to restrict eating would be successful to the point of courting danger.

Understanding the anorectic risk pattern disclosed by our research might begin with a social variable, femininity, with its traditional priority assigned to physical beauty. In the United States and most western cultures, female physical beauty places heavy emphasis upon bodily thinness. Holding physical beauty as a value is important within my proposed explanation of anorectic development, since it would make it more likely that physical appearance would assume priority as the woman redirects her motivation toward a substitute goal. Femininity would not only divert attention toward physical thinness when other goals appear out of reach, but it would continue to lend motivation to food restraint as decreasing weight satisfies the at-risk woman's values regarding bodily attractiveness. To round out the multiple contributions of femininity, a feminine identity would have also contributed to the achievement problems that made goal substitution seem necessary in the first place. Achievement in a professional or social sense, to the extent it is predicated upon competition, presents difficulties for the expressive feminine woman. She is behaviorally predisposed to social transactions that promote reciprocal harmony and not self-centered efforts to compete for contested goals. Problems with competition, misplaced standards, and interpersonal distrust go a long way in explaining the burden of stress found for the at-risk woman that seems to fuel a shift in goal priorities.

The preponderance of personality risk variables for anorexia nervosa that were uncovered are cognitive in nature. Our research disclosed a diverse coalition of cognitive traits, most capable of contributing in a direct and obvious way to the dynamics of food restraint and, thus, to anorectic risk. Repression, a processing variable, was an exception. The tendency for the at-risk woman to selectively forget distressing information would contribute by compromising her problem-solving ability. Repression would make it more likely that she would ignore the problems that precipitated goal substitution; just as femininity contributed to achievement problems, repression hinders their resolution. Furthermore, we cannot ignore the continuing role of repression in anorectic development. The process of body-thinning, once started, would not be effectively challenged as a dysfunctional substitute and a source of new problems by the at-risk female if challenge involved confronting distressing information. Her style is to shunt such information aside and out of consciousness.

Perception, the woman's subjective interpretation of reality, conveniently aligned itself with the at-risk woman's need to achieve thinness. Body image was distorted in the direction of unrealistic fatness which would mean that her quest for thinness remains unsatisfied and her motivation to continue food restraint is sustained. Perceiving her body in such a way as to promote motivation to diet was especially apparent for at-risk women who were thinner to begin with. These women, for whom food restraint is a less realistic option, are most in need of distorted body perception in order to initiate and sustain the dieting process.

Perceptual distortion also serves to solidify resolve for food restraint in another way. Exposure to food cues resulted in an unrealistic sense of body fattening for the vulnerable woman in several studies, and this proved true whether other women's bodies or her own were being considered. The at-risk woman not only places priority on a thin body and distorts her body image to make this goal unattainable, but she adds further to her body distortion in the presence of food cues. It is little wonder that eating would become an especially threatening venture for the at-risk woman obsessed with thinness. Her body already registers perceptually as fatter than it is and then becomes further distended by contemplating food cues. These are not the same phenomenon; our evidence suggested that they contribute to anorectic risk independently of each other.

We also confirmed that the at-risk woman puts herself in a better position to diet successfully because of these perceptual distortions, making more frequent and effective reference to her body size as a dieting strategy. The evidence showed, then, that the at-risk woman not only allows her motivational needs to be served by perceptual distortion, but she puts these distortions to good use as a strategy in her dieting regimen.

An attentional mechanism also was identified as a collaborator in successful eating restraint when at-risk females were found to be less aware of hunger sensations and less responsive to them even if they are recognized. Decreased sensitivity to routine inner sensations signaling hunger would certainly make it easier to avoid eating. Women at anorectic risk were not found to be inattentive to other bodily sensations, so we can assume that the deficit in attention to hunger sensations results from their need to avoid eating. In another analysis, at-risk females reported turbulent levels of inner stimulation, seemingly contributed largely by the emotions of stress that helped define their at-risk status. This inner turbulence may, in fact, contribute to the limited sensitivity reported by these females to hunger sensations. Hunger cues could be lost in the more powerful stimulus milieu provided by stress sensations. This cannot be the whole story, however, since attention to other specific types of inner stimulation was not found lacking in the woman most vulnerable to anorexia nervosa. Whether she shows a specific lack of attention to hunger sensations or these sensations otherwise tend to be lost in a sea of other internal stimulation, some of the insensitivity must represent self-induced denial that abets her need not to eat.

If the many quirks of perception and attention that contribute to food restraint were not enough, aberrant cognition further expands vulnerability to anorexia nervosa through increased self-preoccupation. This cognitive function seems to combine both attentional and perceptual elements as the self-preoccupied woman directs attention toward herself and interprets experiences in egoistic terms. Self-preoccupation in the woman who runs the risk of a future anorectic disorder is hardly surprising in light of her paramount concern about her body and the effects of food upon it. However, our empirical findings regarding this variable suggest that heightened egocentrism takes the woman well beyond an interest in her body proportions and represents a more dynamic part of the risk picture. Intense self-preoccupation may go a long way in distinguishing the vulnerable woman from the woman who values bodily thinness, is a serious dieter, but is not at much risk of anorexia nervosa. Keep in mind that excessive self-reference predisposing the female to continuous concern about herself, especially her body, would magnify the number of occasions when the at-risk woman considered her body image, the perils of eating, compared her body with those of other women, and entertained concerns about how others viewed her appearance. Anorectic risk escalates as the woman is propelled beyond widely-held values regarding size and weight to an obsession with thinness.

The research program into anorectic risk for college women was not only directed toward the psychological variables that characterized the vulnerable female, but it also included some effort to distinguish between the risk for anorexia nervosa and bulimic risk. There are many who believe that these two eating problems are part of the same disorder based primarily on the fact that both may appear in the clinical history of the same woman. I was interested in seeing whether the two abnormal eating patterns associated with weight concerns, the excessive restraint of anorexia nervosa and restraint interspersed with lapses into eating binges and purging of bulimia, could be distinguished at the risk stage.

Considering that so few studies were committed to this end, the results turned out to be rather illuminating. At least, we were able to show that two cognitive parameters of binging were present in college women selected as more at-risk for bulimia; neither was found for college women at greater anorectic risk. Those who were vulnerable to bulimia, as gauged by subclinical symptoms, demonstrated a deficit in self-control which would help explain several aspects of the bulimic disorder -- the failure to satisfy weight concerns by effective dieting, lapses into unrestrained eating, and the failure to curb excessive food intake once a binge begins. Other data showed women at-risk for bulimia to be less attentive to satiety cues that signal fullness and should terminate eating in the normal course of events. Put these self-control and satiety-cue findings together, it becomes easier to understand the unusual phenomenon of binge eating in women who otherwise show concern about food consumption and weight gain. They help explain how binging starts (poor self-control), why it continues (poor self-control), and why it does not stop at some earlier point (poor self-control and disattention to satiety cues).

Although these two sets of findings do not answer all the questions about distinct risk for eating disorders in young-adult college women, they encourage me to believe that anorectic risk can be considered independently of bulimic vulnerability at this point in the genesis of disorder. Why seemingly independent risk for anorexia nervosa and bulimia evolves into alternating disorders in the same woman for some and only one type of eating problem is found in others cannot be answered definitively at this stage of my research. Changes in salience for any of the personality risk factors we have studied could be responsible, but so could any number of psychological factors that we did not study. Broad-based longitudinal research is needed that can trace the growth and changes in psychological risk factors that have been disclosed in our research and others that were not subject to investigation. There is one thread of evidence within the anorectic-risk data that might warrant examination when follow-up investigation is instituted, however.

The woman at anorectic risk displayed several cognitive mechanisms -- styles of cognition that serve the individual's motivational needs --that contributed to eating restraint. These included a body-image distortion that motivates continued dieting, further body-image distortion in response to food cues, and attentional deficit in response to hunger sensations. These cognitive mechanisms almost certainly must be instigated by the at-risk woman's desire not to eat in order to lose weight. We did uncover two additional pieces of evidence suggesting that these cognitive mechanisms may be activated to serve an overriding motivation for thinness.

At-risk women reported that stress resulted in an increase in hunger, whereas other women tended to experience a drop in hunger when stressed. Since stress is a trademark feature of vulnerable females, the increment in hunger that would be expected represents a serious threat to dieting plans in which so much is invested. All of the cognitive mechanisms could have been fomented by the practical necessity of neutralizing increased appetite or deterring an eating relapse by the at-risk woman under stress. She needs all the help she can get and her cognitive functions comply with her wishes. Our research findings also consistently identified the already thinner woman as more at-risk because she combined early symptoms of the disorder, greater amounts of stress, and also revealed one of the perceptual mechanisms being discussed -- body-image distortion. It seemed reasonable to assume that perceptual distortion was required by these thinner women to convince themselves that dieting was required in the first place.

It is when you put these two pieces of evidence side by side that an unusual relationship between them can be noted. Perceptual body-image distortion that promotes food restraint in the thinner woman is geared to arouse stress; the woman obsessed by thinness is bound to be discomforted by an unrealistically fat body. This stress, in turn, increases hunger and threatens food restraint. Increased hunger requires disattention to its sensations and encourages further perceptual distortion of the body image and more stress; etc. Body-image distortion, then, seems to play a paradoxical role in anorectic risk. It facilitates dieting, but at the same time it threatens eating restraint by its likely arousal of stress. This opens the way for distinguishing in some measure between anorectic and bulimic risk at any given point in time by the presence or absence of any of the constituents of this cognitive paradox -- a body on the thinner side, a tendency to perceptually distort body image, heightened stress, and a tendency to experience greater hunger when under stress. Each of these ingredients is subject to wide individual differences and variation over time. Distinguishing between anorectic and bulimic risk for different individuals or within the clinical history of the same individual may depend in some measure upon whether such subtle cognitive patterns are in place to assist symptom development.

I previously offered some suggestions regarding the treatment of college women who show themselves to be at anorectic risk during the preclinical state of the disorder based upon the dynamics of stress alone. Perhaps the clearest implication regarding intervention that I can derive from the added personality-stress interaction risk findings in this section, however, has less to do with how to intervene than with the difficulty of doing so. If the construction I have imposed on the evidence is correct, therapy will face considerable difficulties even at the early risk stage of development. For one thing, professional intervention must contend with a system of traits that complement each other without allowing much in the way of realistic environmental input. Since cognitive mechanisms work in such a way as to more readily achieve food restraint, revising these risk-provoking traits must contend not only with their insulation from reality-testing but also with their functional value in the woman's quest for thinness. Self-preoccupation already serves to intensify these risk factors, at least those associated with body distortion. Intervention may only make the at-risk woman even more self-preoccupied and matters worse.

I would anticipate that the complex motivational role of stress that I proposed would present even greater therapeutic problems if intervention begins deeper into the risk stage of anorectic development. I earlier emphasized two motivational contributions of stress. One was a drive function in which stress energizes woman's striving toward a substitute goal of thinness, and the other was a drive-reduction role in which behaviors that are associated with food restraint and decrease stress, if only momentarily, are strengthened. Now I have proposed a third possibility for the way in which stress may contribute to symptom development. Increments in stress may promote cognitive mechanisms of food restraint by augmenting hunger, challenging the woman's dietary resolve, and compelling even greater distortions of reality to keep from eating. It seems likely that the longer the college female has been caught up in an anorectic progression, the more firmly entrenched would be these varied dynamics of stress.

Given the many ways in which the emotions of stress may influence symptom development, the role of stress might appear to be a reasonable place to concentrate therapeutic efforts. It should be remembered, however, that stress had important origins in the normal striving for career and social goals that ran aground. The at-risk female has already demonstrated her inability to compete for career and social goals, at least in her own eyes, and has been plagued by stress for her also-ran status. It may not be enough to dissuade the at-risk woman from pursuing a thin body as her main priority in order to reinstate standard achievement goals as a way of combatting current stress. The problem of stress would continue unless there was a major psychological modification of her self-defeating approach to conventional goal attainment.

Finally, intervention must contend with the seeming fact that the at-risk female may not want input from the outside as she proceeds towards her goal of body thinness. In fact, she has established the risky progression as a way of reducing her dependency on outside input that has become unwelcome, in part because it is likely to confirm that she falls short of her perfectionistic standards and partly because it is tainted by interpersonal distrust. The more insular goal of achieving thinness has been chosen in no small measure because it offers her some protection from unwelcome intrusion and control. The professional's efforts at evaluation and help may represent more of the same intrusive control.

Stress Dynamics and Stress-Personality Interaction in Menstrual Risk

I already have commented on the limited amount of evidence that was gathered regarding the psychological risk factors in premenstrual syndrome and dysmenorrhea and how this was dictated by research time restraints. It was worth including the results of this line of research, however, because doing so also provided an opportunity to expand upon the dynamic role of stress and how it may compromise biological integrity. Examination of at least a few psychological risk variables accomplished something else as well. Menstrual dysfunctions are the least likely of the three types of psychobiological disorders that were investigated to emphasize psychological risk factors. The role of biological causation in the disorders of menstruation seems evident, and it is the contribution of psychological factors (including stress) that requires verification. The fact that several personality variables emerged as significant in our research with so little investigatory effort affirms the importance of psychological risk as well.

Stress dynamics. Stress was assigned two, possibly three, motivational roles in the risk picture for anorexia nervosa. Stress generates enough unpleasant affect and distracting mentation that it encourages the person to eliminate its aversive presence. This drives the at-risk female toward a new goal that promises satisfactions that have eluded her before and greater freedom from stress. Transitory reductions in stress provided by food avoidance and weight loss strengthen her eating restraint when drive reduction reinforces the system of traits that help the at-risk woman's efforts at dieting. The tendency for stress to increase hunger in the at-risk woman poses a threat to her resolve, however, and compel her to develop or augment cognitive mechanisms that deter eating.

None of these motivational roles assigned to stress makes sense when introduced into the dynamics of women who suffer menstrual dysfunction and are at-risk for even more serious disorder. One good reason for this is that the dysfunctional aspects of the menstrual cycle do not involve any obvious instrumental (goal-oriented) behavior that requires motivation to drive it or must depend upon periodic drive-reduction to sustain it. The dieting behavior of the at-risk anorectic and the competitive achievement-striving of the at-risk Type A both involve instrumental behaviors that require motivational explanation. The pain and anguish of the premenstrual syndrome and dysmenorrhea lack any goal-oriented behavior that I can see, and stress has nothing instrumental to propel by its presence nor to reinforce by its absence.

The symptoms of menstrual dysfunction and the symptoms of stress, as we measured them, offer some degree of similarity both in a physical and a psychological sense. It seems possible that if a woman were being subjected to menstrual problems and to the effects of some stressor at the same time, the two sets of symptoms would tend to combine into a pattern of malaise in which the symptoms would be difficult to distinguish. Since experiencing menstrual dysfunction or even anticipating its arrival can be the basis for generating stress, without even considering other sources in the woman's life, it would be surprising if the discomfort were not often a combination of the two.

This reasoning has led me to propose that PMS and problems during menstrual flow are stress-related disorders and that stress renders its effects in one of two ways. Stress may add its symptoms to those of menstrual dysfunction thereby contributing to the total amount of discomfort or pain experienced by the woman. Either that or stress may sensitize the woman so that her threshold for discomfort and pain is reduced, and she is less able to tolerate the symptoms of menstrual dysfunction. Reduced tolerance would increase the subjective level of distress within the menstrual cycle. It is quite possible, even likely, that these effects of stress are not mutually exclusive. Stress may work in both ways, compounding menstrual symptoms and reducing tolerance for these changes, to increase premenstrual or menstrual dysfunction.

Stress-personality interaction. Despite the limited evidence in hand from our risk research bearing upon menstrual dysfunction, it is possible to make a promising start in piecing together how personality interacts with stress to further compromise this psychobiological system. My proposal for understanding how stress and personality interface in the menstrual risk process is constrained by two things. I am committed to the theoretical framework that guides all three of our research programs, especially the idea that stress of sufficient intensity to place the college female at-risk for stress-related disorder derives in large measure from competitive goal-striving within career and social domains. Accordingly, it is important to relate the evidence concerning menstrual risk to the stress of achievement striving. This is much easier when vulnerability for the other stress-related disorders is being considered, since proposals regarding goal substitution in anorectic risk and competitive striving in the Type A case are conceptually aligned with achieving.

The second constraint results from having to explain why stress affects the menstrual cycle rather than introducing its unwelcome psychobiological effects in another way. This is where the symbolic qualities of the system -- its association with impregnation and childbearing -- serve an explanatory purpose. It is safe to assume that discomfort in varying degrees is commonplace during the menstrual cycle for biological reasons. However, certain women are psychologically less well prepared for these symptoms and react adversely. The greater the rejection of menstrual changes, the more likely stress will be generated to augment that from other sources. The infusion of stress symptoms into the otherwise aversive menstrual changes would only make matters worse for the woman. Since a reduction in tolerance for menstrual symptoms may be part of the rejection, increased sensitivity could magnify augmented menstrual symptoms even further. Acceptance or rejection of menstrual changes has much to do with the symbology of menstruation, or so many have proposed.

The four pieces of evidence regarding the contribution of personality to menstrual dysfunction and the risk of more serious disorder concerned gender-role, role conflict, self-preoccupation, and style of defense against distressing information. Gender-role was the most complicated finding, and I will start there. Our research revealed that if you consider both the actual behaviors of the college woman and her gender-related values or attitudes, the traditional (feminine) and contemporary (masculine) sex-role distinction takes on new meaning. Many college women demonstrate a consistency in these aspects of role behavior; included here would be feminine-behaving women who also hold traditional values and masculine-behaving women who favor contemporary values that emphasize diminished distinctions from men. Perhaps less obvious to popular view, there are many other college females who mix femininity with contemporary attitudes or masculinity with traditional attitudes. I have not collected evidence regarding consistency in role behavior and role attitudes in male college students nor seen it reported elsewhere. This gender-role phenomenon may or may not be important when men are considered.

Role-attitude/role-behavior inconsistency, in defiance of classical clinical thinking regarding conflict and distress, was not associated with premenstrual and menstrual discomfort. The women who were consistent in their commitment to both traditional female role behavior and traditional values showed themselves to be at-risk as they reported greater dysfunction both during the premenstrual period and during actual menstruation. Similarly, consistency between masculine role behavior and contemporary (traditionally male) attitudes also placed the woman at risk for PMS and dysmenorrhea.

Role-conflict evidence, when added to these sex-role results, contributes to understanding menstrual risk as it relates to high stress levels. Role conflict refers to the perceived incompatibility between future career success for the woman and a satisfying marital/childrearing opportunity. This conflict, when assessed in college women, varies enormously. However, it is especially strong in women who combine traditional feminine role behaviors and attitudes, almost nonexistent in women who combine masculinity and contemporary values in a consistent blend, and falls somewhere between for more inconsistent females. Perceived role conflict, then, could serve as a source of stress for the consistently feminine and traditional female. Even more stress should be expected for the woman assuming this kind of homogeneous feminine role from the competitive demands of college matriculation given her expressive orientation. This woman not only behaves in a caring way toward others but endorses the value of expressive transaction. Neither is recommended for effective competitiveness.

A different case must be made for the masculine, contemporary college female based upon the role-conflict results. Not at all concerned about a future conflict between career and marriage, she seems well-prepared for the instrumental, aggressive aspects of competition and achievement. She can concentrate upon career success without being distracted by concern over whether there will be a social price to pay. Distress during the menstrual cycle under these conditions would represent an especially unwelcome and ironic reminder of the symbolic meaning of this biological function. Marriage and children seems to hold no immediate priority, yet she must suffer from a dysfunctional system that prepares her for conceiving children. Upset promoted by the anticipation and actuality of menstrual changes would be only part of the stress picture for the masculine/contemporary college woman, however. The social problems that uncompromising masculinity in the college woman can generate might be expected to contribute their share of stress. The array of socially-alienating traits that distinguished mas-culine and competitive Type A women leads me to expect poor social efficacy in this especially masculine group of women as well. While these college females may not be particularly concerned about a conflict between career opportunities and future marriage at this stage of their lives, that does not mean that they would be impervious to discord in current peer relationships.

If homogeneous gender-roles introduce the risk of premenstrual/menstrual distress through increases in stress, it follows that a more balanced gender-role offers some immunity for American college women in the 1980s and 1990s. Women who temper possible excesses in one aspect of gender-role adoption with somewhat opposing and compensating inclinations in another aspect seem to show a role balance that works in their favor, at least as far as menstrual risk is con-cerned. If this conclusion has a familiar ring to it, there is an echo of androgyny here. The behavior of androgynous women, who attracted considerable scientific and literary attention in the 1970s and 1980s, was thought to be a blend of masculinity and femininity. This blend presumably made her capable of demonstrating a more flexible array of behaviors and to dealing effectively with a more varied assortment of situational demands. Efforts to substantiate the adaptive value of androgyny by rigorous research were not particularly successful despite the popularity of the concept and its convenient place in feminist doc-trine. Perhaps, however, we were emphasizing the wrong blend of mas-culinity and femininity. Rather than demonstrating either type of sex-role behavior depending upon situational requirements, the effective androgyne may combine a predominance of one type of gender-related behavior and the values associated with the opposite gender-role. A softened instrumental character or toughened expressiveness may be what advantageous androgyny is all about, at least in the college woman.

The complications of gender-role and role-conflict explanations of menstrual risk stand in stark contrast to the simplicity of the next risk factor that our research disclosed. Self-preoccupation, already identified as important in explaining the body concern shown by the woman at anorectic risk, also was apparent in the personality risk pat-tern associated with menstrual disorders. If the woman is self-preoccupied, she places herself in a position to respond in full measure to the distress promoted by the combination of menstrual changes and stress. The dynamic timing of self-preoccupation with respect to premenstrual/menstrual distress cannot be established in our research, but most likely it both anticipates the occurrence of aversive monthly changes and follows from the distress that these symptoms bring about. If the woman is more self-preoccupied as she approaches the part of her menstrual cycle when she routinely experiences distress and pain, greater self-awareness would be expected to lower the threshold at which menstrual symptoms register as discomforting. Increments in self-preoccupation that follow the onset of menstrual problems would put a spotlight of attention upon the somatic and behavioral symptoms and magnify their intensity. In either case, self-preoccupation would not only make the distress of menstrual changes worse by lowering tolerance thresholds but also would be responsible for augmenting stress derived from the menstrual cycle as more intense discomfort is anticipated or experienced. The risk of serious premenstrual or menstrual disorder is increased as stress effects are mingled with the distressing symptoms of the dysfunctional biological system.

Circularity of effect seems clearly evident when the role of self-preoccupation in promoting menstrual risk is examined. As seems equally true for risk-induction in anorexia nervosa and Type A-related cardiovascular problems, self-preoccupation can both contribute to the strength of risk-provoking symptoms and derive strength from the symptoms that it helps provoke. I have offered the opinion earlier in this book that self-preoccupation should attract special concern as a risk factor in stress-related disorder, although I may have emphasized its possible contribution to the evolution of other cognitive risk factors. The ease of conceptualizing the circular role of self-preoccupation for all three disorders that we studied adds further to the apparent importance of its psychopathogenic role. Self-preoccupation may turn the attention of the woman toward body thinning in the anorectic risk picture and, in turn, be enhanced by the woman's growing concern about her body and the effects of eating; increases in self-preoccupation would set the stage for ever more obsessive body concerns; etc. By the same token, self-preoccupation may direct the Type A toward competition as she concentrates on egoistic needs, but the failure to satisfy conflicted needs in competition may only intensify self-focus. Circularity of effect in menstrual risk may be the most evidence of all as self-preoccupation increases symptom severity, and symptom severity makes the woman even more self-preoccupied.

The final risk factor found to be associated with menstrual dysfunction involved the woman's defensive style. The findings here were unusual, at least for our research programs, in that the presence of a particular defense pattern qualified as a source of reduced vulnerability to a particular disorder rather than suggesting increased risk. Those who made greater use of rationalization as a protection against otherwise stress-provoking information and did so with minimal awareness of their distortions reported little in the way of premenstrual or menstrual symptoms. There was precedent in earlier investigations of defensive style in college students for this result as the effectiveness of rationalization, especially without awareness, in containing stress was apparent just as repression was confirmed as the poorest defense as far as stress containment was considered. The question remains, however, why unconscious rationalization emerged as a significant counterrisk factor when we studied warning signs for premenstrual and menstrual disorders, whereas unconscious repression assumed importance as a risk indicator for the other stress-related disorders.

I already have offered one possible answer to this question in the chapter on menstrual risk. The biological inevitability of the menstrual cycle and the likelihood of recurring malaise may pose a special challenge to defensive cognition that cannot be resolved very well by being evasive. Effective (stress reducing) short-term protection from the reality of problems that appear inevitable and recurrent might best be derived from acknowledging that the problem actually exists but assigning some meaning or implication that puts it in a more favorable light. It would not be surprising to find that a good many other biological realities are effectively defended by unconscious rationalization -- a body that is too short, heavy, or otherwise deviant from social norms; health that is less that optimal; preference for being of the opposite sex.

Yet there is a special quality to menstrual functioning that may overdetermine why rationalization without awareness could serve as a deterrent to serious problems within the menstrual cycle. The biological importance of the menstrual cycle would be readily apparent for the young college woman entering adulthood. Even if her plans for the foreseeable future did not include marriage, pregnancy, and childrearing, I would think that few college women would choose to deny the importance of these alternatives sooner or later in their adult years. If menstrual functioning not only has an inevitable ring to it but in principle represents a valued asset, the requirements of effective rationalization would be more readily satisfied. The woman should find it less difficult to tolerate distress associated with a biological system that could be convincingly rationalized as necessary at some point in her life.

If intervention in the risk phase of menstrual disorders is attempted, the research evidence suggests that the professional will have to deal with the complicated interface of motivational goals and conflict represented in women at gender-role extremes. The uncertainties involved in role conflict for the purely feminine woman and the frustration of the purely masculine woman with dysfunctional menstruation and a halting social life seem like places to start. In dealing with menstrual risk, you also have to contend with an understandable but maladaptive tendency for afflicted females to be more self-preoccupied. The maladaptive role of self-preoccupation, in turn, provides the same dilemma that confronts therapeutic intervention in every stress-related disorder for which we have explored risk. How do you mitigate self-preoccupation within a therapeutic endeavor that requires the woman's preoccupation with her own personal problems?

Another dilemma that faces intervention in premenstrual/menstrual dysfunction is determining how much of the problem is biological and how much is psychological. Until that is better resolved, the relative importance of medical treatment or psychological intervention remains unclear; as is undoubtedly standard practice now, both therapeutic approaches in liaison are probably warranted. This does not appear to be true when anorectic and Type A risk are considered even though psychobiological disorders are at stake. Medical responsibility for physical symptoms would follow a period, perhaps a very long period, during which psychological risk factors are in need of attention and before the body begins to capitulate to serious life-threatening disorder.

Since dysfunction within the menstrual cycle is generally conceded to be associated with two distinguishable phases of the reproductive system, we routinely studied risk factors independently for the premenstrual period and the period of menstrual flow. The most conservative verdict, given so few studies, would be that the gender-role, defensive style, and self-preoccupation factors are associated with risk for both PMS and dysmenorrhea. If risk seemed more evident for one stress-related disorder or the other, it would be for PMS. Self-preoccupation was more clearly linked to stress in college women reporting distressing symptoms concentrated in the week before menstrual flow, although gender-role and defense as vulnerability factors appeared in the risk picture for both PMS and dysmenorrhea.

Stress Dynamics and Stress-Personality Interaction in Type A Risk

The third series of studies into the risk of psychobiological disorder in college women allowed the most direct examination of the premises underlying all of our stress-and-disorder research and the explanatory context within which the three bodies of evidence are lodged. As the reader will recall, I have assumed that competitive striving toward lofty career goals and social accomplishment at an age when ultimate success or failure remain uncertain is a critical source of stress for the college-age female. Risk for disorder, in turn, is established by the intensity of stress along with the cognitive and social personality traits of the woman that channel stress effects in ways that could prove biologically harmful. Previously-discussed searches for risk factors in anorexia nervosa and premenstrual/menstrual disorders have considered the importance of achievement-striving and competitiveness more by inference than by direct examination. I have had considerable confidence in these assumptions simply because of the subject population that has been the object of study. The typical 18-year-old female college undergraduate in contemporary America is highly motivated to achieve and willing to pit herself against her peers to do so. Some college women are better suited to competition and less conflicted in their goals than others, however.

The Type A personality epitomizes competitive achievement-striving, and these individuals often report the high level of stress that would be expected from their hard-charging ways. The Type A research also provided an opportunity to make empirical comparisons between college females and males in the evidence bearing upon CHD risk. Gender comparisons provide, at the least, a test of whether results can be replicated -- whether findings for one set of individuals can be duplicated when another set is examined. Of greater importance, the comparisons across gender allow me to draw additional conclusions regarding the detrimental long-range effects of stressful ambition upon cardiovascular integrity. Does the risk for the woman match that of the man? At one time, at least, the hard-driving individual who over-commits to success and eventually suffers from heart problems was a male stereotype.

In considering our own Type A research program, I am struck by the amount of measurement refinement that was necessary to make progress in investigating risk. A number of personality variables beyond the basic Type A pattern were found to influence level of stress once these refinements were introduced. It is little wonder that this line of research appears to have fallen short of its early promise. The limited predictiveness of Type A status in studies of cardiovascular risk can be seen as an inevitable consequence of too little concern about what makes the Type A pattern stressful and whether, indeed, it promotes stress at all in many cases. Too little priority was given to questions such as which among the commonly-understood Type A traits are most conducive to stress? Which companion traits compound the intensity of stress? Is stress a problem at all for a given Type A?

Perhaps it is time to resurrect interest in this stress-promoting pattern but with a difference. There should be greater acknowledgement of Type As who do not prove to be heavily stressed and should not be vulnerable to CHD, at least not from chronic activation of the sympathetic nervous system. These are not simply false-positive measurement errors. Lacking the special risk-provoking traits, this benign Type A pattern might even qualify as beneficial for those valuing goals open to competition.

Stress dynamics. Stress was viewed as contributing to risk in quite different ways when anorexia nervosa and menstrual disorders were being considered. I proposed that stress, at least the emotional component, served motivational purposes in anorectic risk by energizing the pursuit of a thin body, reinforcing behaviors that lessen its aversive impact, and further encouraging the adoption of cognitive mechanisms because it increases hunger. Menstrual risk was tied to stress in a very different way as the emotions of stress combine with the dysfunctional symptoms before or during menstruation or decrease the woman's tolerance for these symptoms. In the case of cardiovascular risk, the stress associated with Type A status most likely serves as a pathogenic agent by strenuous and continuing activation of the autonomic nervous system. This could have a "wear-and-tear" effect upon a healthy circulatory system, as Selye (1976) has proposed, or may pose a special danger for those who have some type of preexisting biological vulnerability within the system. Three different risk pictures and three distinct portrayals of the way in which stress can make psychobiological disorder more likely.

A moment's consideration might lead you to question why stress was not treated as serving the same motivational role in Type A risk as it was in anorectic risk. As I mentioned earlier in the book, both anorectic and Type A risk involve instrumental (goal-directed) behaviors that require motivational push and reward. If pursuit of a thin body can be promoted by stress and food restraint rewarded by temporary reductions in stress, why cannot competitive engagement be enhanced in much the same way? As a matter of fact, the role of stress might have been conceived in drive and reinforcement terms if risk of becoming a Type A woman had been subject to explanation. Rather, the long-term effects of stress on the cardiovascular system in Type A individuals was emphasized.

There is no reason, in fact, why stress could not contribute to CHD risk for the Type A in any number of ways. Stress could contribute to Type A personality development, although this remains unstudied in our research. Once the Type A pattern is in place, stress could mobilize the competitive, time-urgent striving that serves as its trademark. Momentary stress reduction that rewards and strengthens traits within the Type A pattern may result from successful achievement along the way, a further motivational effect. Even the conflictual pursuit of respect and liking through aggressive competitive efforts is bound to hit its mark occasionaly for the at-risk Type A woman given enough competitive exposure. This kind of intermittent reinforcement, where egoistic needs are met and tensions drop temporarily, may be enough to maintain the at-risk Type A pattern and its companion traits despite their dysfunctional qualities. All in all, I would say that the contribution of stress to risk provocation plays its most diverse role in the case of cardiovascular problems. The long-range corrosive effects of stress were emphasized, because they related most directly to the risk of CHD as a psychobiological disorder. More immediate motivational effects of stress upon components of the Type A pattern, eventually responsible for CHD, were assumed but not made explicit.

Stress-personality interaction. The substantial number of risk factors that were identified for the vulnerable Type A woman were broken down into three categories. This helped in the conceptualization of Type A risk for me and in the selection of new variables to study. Hopefully it offers a clearer exposition of results for the reader. I focused primarily upon the stress-provoking nature of competition, the hallmark of Type A status, and upon what might influence the amount of stress that would be encountered. These categories of behavior included those that would explain the at-risk Type A's frequent exposure to arousal of stress, the escalation of stress once aroused, and the maintenance of stress over an extended period of time. The arousal and augmentation factors would be used to explain current high stress levels. The maintenance factors are better suited to explaining why this level of stress should persist from the time of investigation until manifest CHD problems appear later in life.

Although convenient for conceptualization and exposition, I have acknowledged that assignment of risk factors to these explanatory categories is to some extent arbitrary. A personality variable verified as a risk factor may have been incorporated in one functional category for sake of exposition, but a rationale could readily be provided for its inclusion in another. Perhaps I am making too much of this conceptual blueprint, since the basic requirement for each variable to qualify as a risk factor was satisfied -- its association with Type A status and elevated stress. Nevertheless, I have made an effort to go beyond stark identification of risk factors in this book by offering some explanation for why each contributed to vulnerability for disorder. Accordingly, I am bothered by acknowledged conceptual blurring, even though some reassurance is derived from the fact that any given trait serves more than one function in complex human behavior. To reiterate the example already given -- there is no reason why a deficit in self-control should not allow more frequent lapses into stressful competition, make it more likely that the Type A will lose restraint and escalate stress for herself while competing, and interfere with efforts on her part to curb competitive zeal over time.

In fact, the extent to which a risk agent could play a diversified role in pathogenesis should mark its importance as a source of vulnerability and as a target for professional intervention. It so happens that flawed self-control qualified conceptually as a multifaceted risk factor for the Type A as well as for women courting bulimic disorder, not so surprising in light of the central problem with restraint observed in both preclinical conditions. Self-preoccupation and sex-role also allowed alternative explanations of risk both within and between stress-related disorders.

Specific risk factors bearing upon control were prominent among • those that would influence whether the Type A woman enters (or creates) stress-arousing competitive situations despite the tension that goes with this kind of interpersonal confrontation. Two different versions of control were identified as mediators of stress. Limited self-control in the Type A female, referring to the ability to regulate her own behavior, was one. The other was an external locus of control of reinforcement, referring to her sense that she does not control the rewards and punishments that may result from her behavior. These control factors suggest a diminished capacity for the at-risk Type A to restrain her competitive inclinations. More than that, any sense that outcomes are not something she can control could encourage the at-risk woman to ignore her mounting history of competitive wins and losses and diminish her motivation to even try. Each contest tends to be a new adventure in competitive striving.

A third risk factor was revealed in the masculinization of the Type A woman. This sex-role orientation would enhance her competitive ways, above and beyond the Type A pattern. The instrumental character of masculinity provides an egoistic goal orientation to build on in which the masculine woman would pursue her own goals with little concern about stepping on some figurative toes along the way. The combination of Type A competitiveness and masculine instrumental qualities would promise a motivated readiness to contest for goals and invite the stress that goes with it. This readiness to compete in masculine Type As, in psychological league with the two control deficits, goes a long way in explaining the hypercompetitiveness that defines stress-prone Type A status in the college woman.

Further disclosures regarding the masculinity of the Type A female point toward stress from other sources as well. On the one hand, personality correlates from two studies revealed a broad array of interpersonal behaviors that augur poorly for social adjustment. When asked to describe their own behavior and these revelations were compared with Type Bs, Type A college women portrayed themselves as more argumentative, cynical, demanding, faultfinding, impatient, opinionated, outspoken, quarrelsome, resentful, touchy, and tough. At the same time, the Type A came out as less appreciative, cheerful, gentle, kind, sincere, thoughtful, tolerant, trusting, unselfish, and warm. With so many annoying to distressing characteristics and so few redeeming qualities appearing in her self-appraisal, the female type A either qualifies as a social misfit or as terribly self-effacing. Presenting a humble facade does not fit well with the at-risk Type A's chosen role as an aggressive competitor; being assertively frank in her self-description is far more likely.

A third study considered Type A gender-role and broader personality traits rather than discrete behavioral characteristics, and the verdict was much the same. At-risk Type A women were depicted as generally masculine in character with traits that would promote independence of others (except for needing emotional gratification) -- extreme aggressiveness, lack of warmth or generosity, a disinclination to be friendly, and insensitivity to the meaning of interpersonal behavior. A rather dismal social picture for the at-risk Type A woman is again suggested. Since far-ranging social problems seem inevitable given this repeated picture of alienating behaviors, I would expect even more stress to be added to the burden created by Type A obsession with achievement through competition.

Sex-role may well add further to stress evocation for the at-risk Type A woman beyond the contribution of her masculine instrumental qualities to competitive fervor and her seemingly abrasive and alienating ways to social ineffectiveness. Masculinity in the at-risk Type A woman, somewhat surprisingly, was accompanied by a well-developed sensitivity to traditional sex-role values. Her masculinity, her Type A aggressive competitiveness and achievement-striving, and her social demeanor seem remarkably out of character with her well-developed sensitivity to traditional role assignments for the woman. While the masculine hypercompetitive and socially-abrasive Type A woman who is at-risk remains cognizant of traditional feminine expectations, I can only assume that she has no intention of conforming to those expectations. Rather, I would expect her to contentiously oppose any effort to force her into the feminine mold, the kind of role she most likely rejects. This may help explain her interpersonal style. The expressive core of traditional femininity resides in harmonious social transactions. Rejection of the expressive orientation would make the disharmonious social style disclosed by research more predictable and seemingly a matter of deliberate choice.

This array of gender-role effects that were revealed by our investigation of stress in the Type A college woman provides a rather remarkable affirmation of this variable in her risk for eventual psychobiological disorders. The sex-role factor proved significant in each of the three programs of research as a correlate of stress, but the variety of ways that sex-role seemed to contribute to stress and the risk it imposes was equally impressive. Masculinity in women was the paramount source of vulnerability in Type A CHD risk, femininity loomed as more important in anorectic risk, and both sex-roles qualified as risk factors when premenstrual/menstrual risk were studied depending upon the presence of corresponding role attitudes. At the same time, what limited comparisons we made with male college students gave no hint that gender role serves as a source of risk. The most evident conclusion is that by the decade of the '90s accommodation to or dismissal of traditional role expectations are still of vital importance to the college woman, but this does not seem to be the case for their male peers.

A second category of risk variables was geared to explaining the singularly stressful nature of competition for the at-risk Type A woman rather than its frequent occurrence. The issue of who will win and who will lose in competition, either in episodic contests that come and go or in long-term pursuit of more substantial goals, provokes stress for most ambitious people. Augmenting risk factors derive their importance from the premise that CHD risk would be enhanced if the Type A brought additional psychological baggage into competition that made it more stress-provoking for her than for other college women. These variables reveal the real dysfunctional core of the at-risk Type A -- unrelenting competitiveness despite its more stressful consequences.

Self-preoccupation again qualified as a risk variable just as had been the case in the other two programs of study into stress-related disorder. Our reasoning was that the egoism implied by self-preoccupation would make the outcome of competition more critical for the Type A woman and the situation more stressful. As the contest is joined, the female Type A is exposed to her compelling ambition for achievement in whatever form and to the importance of competitive outcome to that end. The egoism of the Type A would only make matters worse as far as stress induction is concerned. It could encourage a very low standard for what constitutes legitimate achievement or simply distort the importance of winning.

Another stress-augmenting risk variable in competition may well turn out to be even more critical than simply winning or losing the contest. A two-trait personality pattern shown by the at-risk Type A woman seemed linked to inevitable conflict within a competitive transaction. Despite being remarkably independent in terms of the more obvious behavioral mechanics of personal responsibility, the at-risk Type A female maintains an emotional dependency on others that would be satisfied by receiving outside support, approval, and evidence of likability. At the same time, she presents a picture of being highly aggressive; aggression involves the intention of harm to someone or something. While emotional dependency might be difficult to satisfy given the Type A's rather caustic social demeanor, a need for approval and an aggressive style within competition would be an even less promising combination. Those with whom you aggressively compete are unlikely candidates for satisfying your need for approval and liking. Finding evidence for a stress-promoting conflict within competition offered new insight on the self-preoccupation variable as well. The egoism of the Type A woman that qualified as a risk factor can be tied not only to the woman's concern about winning or losing. At some level she should recognize that her aggressive competitive style is not conducive to satisfying another egoistic concern -- gaining evidence that she is respected or liked by those with whom she is competing.

The final category of risk factors was intended to cast light on the issue of chronicity for the personality characteristics constituting the basic Type A pattern and its correlates, all proposed as risk factors. Some basis for anticipating long-term maintenance of the stress levels they produce was needed. The issue here boils down to the question of whether personality and stress can be projected ahead to a period in life when the cardiovascular system is more likely to finally capitulate to sustained emotional arousal? I might have been able to fall back on the fact that our research defined risk in terms of cognitive and social personality traits which can be presumed to have some degree of stability by 18 years of age. Reasoning this way, the behaviors that invoke stress at a college age will tend to be found as the woman grows older -- once an at-risk Type A, always an at-risk Type A. While I believe that some degree of stability can be expected for female Type A personality and other risk factors, something more in way of explanation seemed required in order to project the long-term continuation of the problem-ridden profile of traits as a conduit for stress. That "something more" involved a number of cognitive skills or styles that would ordinarily contribute to problem-solving ability but were notably absent in the Type A. One good basis for predicting the stability of traits that are conducive to problem behavior and stress is a diminished capacity to solve problems or even recognize that they exist.

The readiness of the Type A woman to identify and resolve personal problems was considered by a number of reanalyses of data collected for other purposes, and these serendipitous findings were followed by planned investigation specifically designed to clarify Type A risk. Preferred defense style was one of the cognitive variables studied through reanalysis -- the manner in which someone alters distressing information as a way of temporarily avoiding its emotional consequences. Type A women made special use of repressive tactics in which distressing information is put out of mind and forgotten, at least until it is resurrected by a compelling reminder. The degree of evasiveness involved in this style of defense is maximum relative to other alternative strategies that distort or simply deny the distressing message. As the Type A woman tries to forget troublesome elements of her problems, problem-solving is likely deferred or ineptly pursued.

Other cognitive variables that qualified as risk factors when file evidence was reexamined had less to do with motivated procrastination than with limitations in recognizing or resolving problems even when the elements of the problem should be apparent. Examination of these social-acuity factors found the Type A woman to be consistently lacking in the activity or skill important to effective problem-solving. Prior data revealed Type A deficits in: (1) intraception, the tendency to think in terms of why people do things rather than what they do; (2) social insight, the ability to appraise the complexities of interpersonal relationships; and (3) facial-decoding skill, the ability to recognize emotions from the facial expressions of others. In addition, the Type A woman was found to have a (4) high tolerance for ambiguity, a seeming reticence to assign meaning to an otherwise unclear stimulus. Tolerating ambiguity not only makes the recognition of a problem more difficult, but, like repression, contributes to procrastination.

The consistent implication from one sample of college women to the next was that being Type A meant falling short in motivation or skill when it comes to problem-solving. The Type A woman would be slow to recognize when a problem exists (poorer facial decoding and a very high tolerance for ambiguity), given to putting problems aside even when they are recognized (repression), and handicapped in problem-solving should she actually make the effort (lower intraception and social insight).

The four social-acuity factors -- intraception, social insight, facial decoding, and tolerance of ambiguity -- were reaffirmed as potential obstacles to problem-solving for Type A women in a follow-up study but with important refinements. I have emphasized the importance of establishing impaired problem-solving in Type As as a way of explaining the chronicity of stress and bridging the time between our research with young-adult college students and CHD symptoms that are most likely to appear later in life. If the personal problems of the Type A persist or new problems defying resolution can be expected, stress chronicity becomes a more reasonable expectation. There is a second reason why poor problem-solving plays an important explanatory role for Type As. Considerable evidence has been uncovered suggesting conflicted motives in competition for Type As who are most at-risk -- emotional dependency and aggressive competitiveness. Why such obvious discord in motivational goals remains unnoticed or at least unresolved as a problem by college age and continues as a source of stress requires explanation. Poor problem-solving provides a reasonable way to understand the recurrence of this conflict. As it turned out, only at-risk Type As who reported a conflict between approval-seeking and aggressiveness within competitive situations were lacking in social acuity, and this proved to be true for both females and males. Other Type As and all Type Bs looked much alike in presenting the higher social acuity that would be expected among intelligent college students. There was evidence in the Heilbrun and Karp study that the coupling of motive conflict and poor problem resolution, although present in both sexes, was a more serious matter for the at-risk woman than for her male counterpart. Only the vulnerable Type A reported excessive stress among the women, whereas at-risk men did not reveal anything extraordinary in the way of stress. Our earlier studies had not disclosed any gender difference in the risk associated with motive conflict in competition.

Perhaps the safest conclusion in light of this irregularity of the evidence is that the motivational conflict may contribute to CHD risk, because it arouses stress and is sustained by poor problem-solving skills in the Type A of either gender. If there is a sex difference, conflicted motives should be considered a more important risk factor for the Type A woman. The fact that gender-role was important in understanding Type A risk-provocation only in the female argues for the possibility that this may be more of a problem for college women. Emotional dependency, a feminine trait, is remarkably out of character with the at-risk Type A woman's masculinity, especially her aggressive competitiveness. It not only results in conflicted motives, but is part of a traditional role she rejects. In the case of Type A college men, the conflicted motives do not appear to be part of a broader picture of sex-role commitment and rejection.

Refinement in problem-solving evidence within the Heilbrun and Karp study also accomplished something else. It examined all four social-acuity factors together in a single body of data so that the results could verify a broadly-based impairment in problem-solving in the same set of at-risk Type A women. Previous evidence calling upon results from several studies revealed isolated social-acuity deficits, with each deficit found in a different sample of college Type As. Confirming the breadth of cognitive problem-solving skills that are below par in a given Type A spares me the necessity of assuming profound deficits of any one type (which were not found). At-risk Type As are lacking in cognitive problem-solving skills in every way possible, at least every way that was examined.

Prospects for professional intervention into a stress-provoking Type

A commitment for the college woman seem to provide room for both optimism and pessimism. On the optimistic side, the sheer number of type-defining and collaborating personality traits that enter into the provocation, augmentation, and maintenance of stress provides a great deal of latitude to the professional. There will be any number of behavioral dispositions that collectively are compromising the quality of the woman's life and placing her at-risk for eventual cardiovascular problems.

Not only are there diverse problematic entry points into the Type A woman's stressful life, but some of the points of intervention involve rather glaring inconsistencies that call out for resolution. These should be obvious to the Type A but probably are not because of her elusive approach to problems and her blunted social acuity. Such self-destructive inconsistencies should be especially profitable places to direct therapeutic attention. Examples here should start with the conflict between emotional dependency and aggressiveness that lends a self-defeating quality to the hallmark competitiveness of the Type A woman. I have given that conflict enough attention, so I will not go through it again. However, there are several other inconsistencies that can be observed within the evidence of risk-provoking Type A behavior that have not been as fully elaborated.

For one, the data revealed that masculinity, which seems to play such a prominent role in both the at-risk Type A female's competitive efforts for achievement and her alienating interpersonal style, is displayed despite retaining her sensitivity to traditional feminine sex-role expectations. Perhaps this is a legacy of feminist commitment as traditional expectations command attention simply because they are so avidly rejected. The inconsistency here is between being masculine, probably very masculine, in her behavioral style and the constant reminder that this option is out of step with tradition. While her masculinity may satisfy her need to adopt a new role for women, her "anything but feminine" mindset would make it more likely the at-risk Type A woman will play out her role in a contentious way. Her seemingly abrasive social style could be the result. As our evidence suggests, Type A masculinity is not conducive to stress if the college woman does not remain sensitive to the issue of cultural tradition.

Yet other inconsistences that would merit therapeutic attention are inherent in the at-risk Type A woman's strong independence, her self-willed preference to do things on her own. As you may recall, this tendency to not lean on others for assistance, suggested by greater autonomy and lesser deference, was distinguished behaviorally from succorance that entails emotional dependency. Inconsistency begins with this distinction between forms of dependency. If the woman is going to be autonomous in her dealings with others, it becomes difficult to position herself socially so as to satisfy her need for emotional support. As I mentioned more than once, attempts to satisfy emotional dependency are peculiarly pursued in the context of aggressive competition; her independence from others helps explain why this odd arrangement may be all the Type A woman has open to her in the absence of immediate family. The independence of the at-risk Type A female also seems curiously out of line with her external locus of control. What sense is there in the independence of the Type A woman that involves assuming responsibility for her own actions if reinforcement outcomes are viewed as being out of her hands?

An abundance and variety of problematic behaviors may qualify the Type A woman as a promising candidate for early intervention during the CHD risk period, but there are indications that difficulties would be encountered that go beyond those that regularly accompany efforts to modify problem behavior in college students. The sheer number of risk factors that identify the at-risk Type A as in need of psychological help also present a quandary for the professional. How do you address your therapeutic efforts when there are so many aspects of personality that feed into this woman's stress? Which critical personality elements -- competitiveness, gender-role, self-preoccupation, self-control, etc. -- provide the glue holding this pattern together? Strategy of intervention assumes paramount importance when the troubled individual has so many disadvantageous psychological dispositions.

The most serious hurdle facing intervention that I can see, however, is the apparent problem that the at-risk Type A female would have in participating constructively in the therapeutic process. So many of the traits that have been documented in our research as contributing to the stress-provoking pattern could be detrimental to her assuming an effective client's role. Her tendency to avoid rather than confront distressing information, to act on her own and not depend on others, to compete aggressively in any way she can, her abrasive transactional style, and especially her limited social acuity could make the Type A something less than an ideal participant in therapy. In fact, the difficulty in rendering help may begin with getting her to seek or accept it in the first place despite the stressful life she leads.

Gender comparison in Type A risk. The comparison of Type A college women to their male counterparts with regard to CHD risk resulted in far more similarities than differences. To begin with, Type As were found to be under considerably higher stress than Type Bs for both sexes. This finding, consistent with Type A theory but not routinely demonstrated in Type A research, was found with such regularity that it frequently went unnoted in the narrative portion of the book. However, the expected contingency between Type A status and stress appeared at compelling levels only when measurement of the basic coronary-prone pattern was revised and additional risk factors were introduced. This observation applies to both sexes as well.

The additional cognitive risk factors that were associated with stress arousal, augmentation, and maintenance in pattern A college students were confirmed uniformly without respect to gender. Most notably, self-control deficit, an external locus of control, all the evidence bearing on the approval-seeking/aggression conflict within competition, repressive defensiveness, and problem-solving limitations emerged as specific risk factors for Type A women and men alike.

The clearest exception to the commonality of Type A risk across gender lines came within the sex-role domain. Sex-role emerged as a more important risk variable for college women than for their male peers. The adoption of a Type A pattern of behavior by a masculine female seems to foster consequences that go well beyond enhancing competitive endeavor; it also seems to diminish the quality of her social transactions in general. The evidence suggests that the masculine at-risk Type A woman has a choice between conflict-ridden competition and other social transactions that are just about as conducive to stress. Nothing comparable emerged in the evidence on Type A risk in college men.

Why sex-role should play a more vital role in Type A risk for the college woman than for the college man is a matter for conjecture. My guess would be that the Type A pattern is a more formidable commitment for the college female than for her male counterpart. Career-related achievement striving and competitiveness along with an eventual marital union remain a cultural legacy for college males without regard to their sex-role identity. Being male means that you are open to all of the psychological risk factors that are associated with Type A excesses and deficits that promote stress, and this is the case whether you are masculine or feminine. College women, however, face a different heritage so that sex-role makes a greater difference in today's world of competitive achievement. Only the masculine woman is likely to take on the behavioral excesses of the Type A pattern as she selectively pursues career success with a vengeance. In contesting what was at one time a preclusive male goal, however, the masculine Type A woman is more likely to overinvest herself, place her social goals in jeopardy, invite serious stress, and increase her risk for CHD.

An Overview of the At-risk Evidence

I suppose the greatest fear that researchers can have, at least those who commit themselves to programmatic research, is that they will come up with nothing worth discussing even by their own analysis. Running a close second is a concern that they will compile a set of results that appear important to them but will simply be ignored; since a brief half-life is the fate of most published research findings in psychology, even that destiny should not come as a surprise. However, there is an understandable temptation at the end of a published summation of research evidence like this to say something that will win the day and better guarantee some impact and a continuing interest in what the evidence suggests. My problem is that I have said almost everything that occurs to me regarding the importance of clarifying the progression into stress-related disorder of college women during the preclinical period of risk and about the at-risk research method by which I attempted to do this. I have fully reported the risk factors that were discovered, and have provided a rationale in each case for their role in arousing stress and creating a vulnerability to disorder. Only a few final thoughts seem to be in order.

I have tried very hard to refrain from specific suggestions concerning what is to be done professionally should risk indicators for stress-related disorder be encountered in young-adult college women. Risk patterns signaling the future danger of anorexia nervosa, menstrual disorders, or CHD have been presented as a source of diagnostic assistance that can more firmly establish whether therapeutic intervention is required to avert disorder and what directions such assistance might take. The choice of method by which behavior is to be modified must depend upon the wisdom of therapists and the skills that they can bring to bear. I would imagine that a range of possibilities might be effective depending upon which risk factor within which progression of disorder is being considered. What might work in modifying the narrowly-focused distorted perceptions contributing to anorectic risk would likely be inadvisable given the complicated sex-role/gender-schema/Type A interaction serving as a source of vulnerability for the female at-risk for CHD.

Those who are interested in the epidemiology of stress-related disorder in women on the college campus may have found the search for risk factors across several disorders to be instructive. The at-risk approach to research not only promises progress toward prediction and prevention on several fronts, but it allows a rare empirical examination of common or distinguishing risk factors across several disorders. The future of understanding stress-provoked vulnerability to psychobiological dysfunction may require us to go beyond the identification of risk factors for just one particular health problem. It may be possible to formulate a profile of vulnerability when college women report a discomforting level of stress that would provide a hierarchy of risk across a variety of disorders. Although our data fall short of realizing this end, they do mark a beginning. As examples of starting points for vulnerability profiles, our evidence suggests that self-preoccupation is common to vulnerability across several disorders and would serve as a warning of multiple risk. At the other extreme, gender-role identity could provide a basis for discriminating risk in college women under stress as femininity, masculinity, and role behavior-role attitude combinations signal different types of vulnerability.

The extent to which the fruits of our research labor will prove valuable in predicting and preventing disorder can be established given its tentative acceptance by the community of professionals concerned with the welfare of young-adult college women. Professional experience can serve as a preliminary jury for the at-risk evidence. Subsequently, longitudinal research that would follow the evolution of disorder from the period of risk into clinical certainty could offer a rigorous test of our findings.

Although I have stopped short of presenting the research evidence in this book as the basis for developmental theories of disorder, I have come close when attempting to cast our risk findings in a meaningful explanatory context. The assumption has been that the risk factors identified by our research would be more compelling if I could go beyond empirical confirmation by statistical test to the further requirement that they make sense as sources of vulnerability to one stress-related disorder or another. Stress itself proved to be a substantial challenge to elaborating a context of understanding for each set of risk variables. It was necessary to call upon a number of functional roles that stress must assume in pathogenesis in order to explain why high stress should play a vital part within the three risk patterns. Now that the evidence is in, there is only one conclusion that can be reached in my opinion. Stress, nurtured by personality, does serve as an important basis for anorexia nervosa, disorders of the menstrual cycle, and Type A-based CHD, and it does so in an alarming number of ways.

References

Abraham, K. (1948). Manifestations of the female castration complex. In K.Abraham (Ed.), Selected papers on psychoanalysis. London: Hogarth.

Adler, A. (1939). The science of living. Garden City, NY: Garden City Publishing Co.

Adorno, T. W., Frenkel-Brunswik, E., Levinson, D.J., & Sanford, R. M. (1950). The authoritarian personality. New York: Harper & Row.

Allen, L. R. (1969). Self-esteem of male alcoholics. Psychological Record, 19, 381-389.

Allen, L. R., & Dootjes, I. (1968). Some personality considerations of an alcoholic population. Perceptual and Motor Skills, 27, 707-712.

American Psychiatric Association: Committee on Nomenclature and Statistics (1987). Diagnostic and statistical manual of mental disorder (DSM-III-R). Washington, D.C.: Author.

Amos, E., & Khanna, P. (1985). Life stress in spasmodic and congestive dysmenorrhea. Psychological Reports, 57, 216-218.

Balint, M. (1937). A contribution to the psychology of menstruation. Psychoanalytic Quarterly, 6, 346-352.

Batlis, N., & Small, A. (1982). Sex roles and Type A behavior. Journal of Clinical Psychology, 38, 315-316.

Bem, S. L. (1981a). Gender schema theory: A cognitive account of sex typing. Psychological Review, 88, 354-364.

Bem, S. L. (1981b). Bem Sex Role Inventory professional manual. Palo Alto, CA: Consulting Psychologists Press.

Benedek, T. (1959). The sexual functions in women. In S. Arieti (Ed.), American handbook of psychiatry. New York: Basic Books.

Berry, C., & McGuire, F. (1972). Menstrual distress and acceptance of sex role. American Journal of Obstetrics and Gynecology, 114, 82-87.

Blake, R. R., & Vanderplas, J. M. (1950). The effect of pre-recognition hypotheses on the veridical recognition thresholds in auditory perception. Journal of Personality, 19, 95-115.

Blane, H. T. (1968). The personality of the alcoholic: Guises of dependency. New York: Harper & Row.

Block, J. (1961). Ego identity, role variability, and adjustment. Journal of Consulting Psychology, 25, 392-397.

Blumenthal, J. A., Williams, R. B., Kong, Y., Schanberg, S. M., & Thompson, L. W. (1978). Type A behavior pattern and coronary atherosclerosis. Circulation, 58, 634-639.

Bransford, J. D., & Franks, J. J. (1971). The abstraction of linguistic terms. Cognitive Psychology, 2, 331-350.

Brattesani, K., & Silverthorne, C. P. (1978). Social psychological factors of menstrual distress. Journal of Social Psychology, 106, 139-140.

Caffrey, B. (1970). A multivariate analysis of sociopsychological factors in monks with myocardial infarction. American Journal of Public Health, 60, 452-457.

Cameron, N. (1963). Personality development and psychopathology: A dynamic approach. Boston: Houghton Mifflin.

Case, R. B., Heller, S. S., Case, N. B., Moss, A. J., & The Multicenter Post-infarction Research Group (1985). Type A behavior and survival after acute myocardial infarction. The New England Journal of Medicine, 312, 737-741.

Charalampous, K. D., Ford, B. K., & Skinner, T. J. (1976). Self-esteem in alcoholics and nonalcoholics. Journal of Studies on Alcohol, 37, 990-994.

Chernovetz, M. E., Jones, W. H., & Hansson, R. O. (1979). Predictability, attentional focus, sex-role orientation, and menstrual-related stress. Psychosomatic Medicine, 41, 383-391.

Clare, A. W. (1979). The treatment of premenstrual symptoms. British Journal of Psychiatry, 135, 576-579.

Crow, T. (1980). Molecular pathology of schizophrenia: More than one disease process? British Medical Journal, 180, 66-68.

Crow, T. J. (1985). The two-syndrome concept: Origins and current status. Schizophrenia Bulletin, 11, 471-486.

Damas-Mora, J., Davies, L., Taylor, W., & Jenner, F. A. (1980). Menstrual respiratory changes and symptoms. British Journal of

Psychiatry, 136, 492-497.

DeGregorio, E., & Carver, C. (1980). Type A behavior pattern, sex role orientation, and psychological adjustment. Journal of Personality and Social Psychology, 39, 286-293.

Dembroski, T. M. (1978). Reliability and validity methods used to assess coronary-prone behavior. In T. M. Dembroski, S. M. Weiss, J. L. Shields, S. G. Haynes, & M. Feinleib (Eds.), Coronary-prone behavior (pp. 95-106). New York: Springer-Verlag.

Deutsch, H. (1944). The psychology of women. New York: Grune & Stratton.

Diller, R. (1986). An examination of the effects of role conflict on young women. Master's thesis, Emory University, Atlanta, Georgia.

Dimsdale, J. E., Hackett, T. P., Hutter, A. M., Block, P. C., & Catanzano, D. M. (1978). Type A personality and extent of coronary atherosclerosis. The American Journal of Cardiology, 42, 583-586.

Dimsdale, J. E., Hackett, T. P., Hutter, A. M., Block, P. C., Catanzano, D. M., & White, P. J. (1979). Type A behavior and angiographic findings. Journal of Psychosomatic Research, 23, 273-276.

Edwards, A. L. (1957). Manual for the Edwards Personal Preference Schedule. New York: Psychological Corporation.

Ekman, P., & Friesen, W. V. (1976). Pictures of facial affect. Palo Alto, CA: Consulting Psychologists Press.

Ekman, P., Friesen, W. V., & O'Sullivan, M. (1977). Reading of facial expressions: A self-test. Kenilworth, NJ: Schering Corporation.

Frederiksen, J. R. (1966). A study of perceptual recognition in two sense modalities. (Research Bulletin 66-32). Princeton, NJ: Educational Testing Service.

Frenkel-Brunswik, R. (1949). Intolerance of ambiguity as an emotional and perceptual personality variable. Journal of Personality, 18, 108-143.

Freud, S. (1911). Psychoanalytical notes on an autobiographical account of a case of paranoia. In J. Strachey (Ed.). S.E., vol. XII. London: Hogarth, 1958.

Freud, S. (1915). Repression. In J. Strachey (Ed.). S.E., vol. XIV. London: Hogarth, 1957.

Freud, S. (1938). Totem and taboo. In A. A. Brill (Ed.), The basic writings of Sigmund Freud. New York: Random House.

Friedman, M., & Rosenman, R. H. (1959). Association of specific overt behavior pattern with blood and cardiovascular findings. Journal of the American Medical Association, 169, 1288-1296.

Friedman, M., & Rosenman, R.(1974). Type A behavior and your heart. New York: Knopf.

Garner, D. M., Olmstead, M. P., & Polivy, J. (1983). Development and validation of a multidimensional eating disorder inventory of anorexia and bulimia. International Journal of Eating Disorders, 2, 15-31.

Good, P. R., & Smith, B.D. (1980). Menstrual distress and sex-role attributes. Psychology of Women Quarterly, 4, 482-490.

Gottesman, I. J., McGuffin, P., & Farmer, A. E. (1987). Clinical genetics as clues to the "eal" genetics of schizophrenia (a decade of modest gains while playing for time). Schizophrenia Bulletin, 13, 23-47.

Gough, H. G. (1965). A validational study of the Chapin Social Insight Test. Psychological Reports, 17, 355-368.

Gough, H. G. (1968). The Chapin Social Insight Test manual. Palo Alto, CA: Consulting Psychologists Press.

Gough, H. G. (1975). Personality factors related to severity of menstrual distress. Journal of Abnormal Psychology, 84, 59-65.

Gough, H. G., & Heilbrun, A. B. (1965). Manual for the Adjective Check List and the need scales for the ACL. Palo Alto, CA: Consulting Psychologists Press.

Gough, H. G., & Heilbrun, A. B. (1980). Manual for the Adjective Check List. Palo Alto, CA: Consulting Psychologists Press.

Grant, D. A., & Berg, E. A. (1948). A behavioral analysis of degree of reinforcement and ease of shifting to new responses in a Weigl-type card-sorting problem. Journal of Experimental Psychology, 38, 404-411.

Greenberg, R. P. & Fisher, S. (1984). Menstrual discomfort, psychological defenses, and feminine identification. Journal of Personality Assessment, 48, 643-648.

Gruba, G. H., & Rohrbaugh, M. (1975). MMPI correlates of menstrual distress. Psychosomatic Medicine, 37, 265-273.

Guy, R. F., Rankin, B. A., & Norvell, B. (1980). The relation of sex role stereotyping to body image. The Journal of Psychology, 105, 167-173.

Haft, M. (1973). An exploratory study of early adolescent girls: Body image, self-acceptance, acceptance of "traditional female role," and response to menstruation. Dissertation Abstracts International, 35, 4173-B.

Hawkins, R. C., Turrell, S., & Jackson, L. J. (1983). Desirable and undesirable masculine and feminine traits in relation to students' dieting tendencies and body image dissatisfaction. Sex Roles, 9, 705-717.

Haynes, S. G., Feinleib, M., & Kannel, W. B. The relationship of psychosocial factors to coronary heart disease in the Framington Study. III. Eight-year incidence of coronary heart disease. American Journal of Epidemiology, 1980, III (1), 37-58.

Heilbrun, A. B. (1959). Validation of a need scaling technique for the Adjective Check List. Journal of Consulting Psychology, 23, 347-351.

Heilbrun, A. B. (1971). Style of adaptation to perceived maternal stimulation and selective attention to evaluative cues. Journal of Abnormal Psychology, 77, 340-344.

Heilbrun, A. B. (1972). Defensive projection in late adolescents: Implications for a developmental model of paranoid behavior. Child Development, 43, 880-891.

Heilbrun, A. B. (1973). Aversive maternal control: A theory of schizophrenic development. New York: Wiley.

Heilbrun, A. B. (1976). Measurement of masculine and feminine sex-role identities as independent dimensions. Journal of Consulting and Clinical Psychology, 44, 183-190.

Heilbrun, A. B. (1977). The influence of defensive styles upon the predictive validity of the Thematic Apperception Test. Journal of Personality Assessment, 41, 486-491.

Heilbrun, A. B. (1978). Projective and repressive styles of processing aversive information. Journal of Consulting and Clinical Psychology, 46, 156-164.

Heilbrun, A. B. (1981a). Human sex-role behavior. New York: Pergamon.

Heilbrun, A. B. (1981b). Gender differences in the functional linkage between androgyny, social cognition, and competence. Journal of Personality and Social Psychology, 41, 1106-1118.

Heilbrun, A. B. (1982a). Psychological scaling of defensive cognitive styles on the Adjective Check List. Journal of Personality Assessment, 46, 495-505.

Heilbrun, A. B. (1982b). Tolerance for ambiguity in female clients: A further test of the catharsis model for predicting early counseling dropout. Journal of Counseling Psychology, 29, 567-571.

Heilbrun, A. B. (1984a). Cognitive defenses and life stress: An information-processing analysis. Psychological Reports, 54, 3-17.

Heilbrun, A. B. (1984b). Sex-based models of androgyny: A further cognitive elaboration of competence differences. Journal of Personality and Social Psychology, 46, 216-229.

Heilbrun, A. B. (1986). Androgyny as type and androgyny as behavior: Implications for gender schema in males and females. Sex Roles, 14, 123-138.

Heilbrun, A. B. (1989). Type A, locus of control, and stress: Another case in point. Psychological Reports, 64, 524-526.

Heilbrun, A. B., & Abraham, J. R. (1987). Psychological complexity of self-control impairment in alcoholism. British Journal of Addiction, 82, 209-210.

Heilbrun, A. B., & Bloomfield, D. L. (1986). Cognitive differences between bulimic and anorexic females: Self-control deficits in bulimia. International Journal of Eating Disorders, 5, 209-222.

Heilbrun, A. B., Blum, N., & Goldreyer, N. (1985). Defensive projection: An investigation of its role in paranoid delusions. Journal of Nervous and Mental Disease, 173, 17-25.

Heilbrun, A. B., Cassidy, J. C., Diehl, M., Haas, M., & Heilbrun, M. R. (1986). Psychological vulnerability to alcoholism: Studies of internal scanning deficit. British Journal of Medical Psychology, 59, 237-244.

Heilbrun, A. B., Diller, R. S., & Dodson, V. S. (1986). Defensive projection and paranoid delusions. Journal of Psychiatric Research, 20, 161-173.

Heilbrun, A. B., & Flodin, A. (1989). Food cues and perceptual distortion of the female body: Implications for food avoidance in the early dynamics of anorexia nervosa. Journal of Clinical Psychology, 45, 843-851.

Heilbrun, A. B., & Frank, M. E. (1989). Self-preoccupation and general stress level as sensitizing factors in premenstrual and menstrual distress. Journal of Psychosomatic Research, 33, 571-577.

Heilbrun, A. B., & Friedberg, E. B. (1987). Type A behavior and stress in college males. Journal of Personality Assessment, 51, 555-564.

Heilbrun, A. B., & Friedberg, E. B. (1988). Type A personality, self-control, and vulnerability to stress. Journal of Personality Assessment, 52, 420-433.

Heilbrun, A. B., & Friedberg, L. (1990). Distorted body image in normal college women: Possible implications for the development of anorexia nervosa. Journal of Clinical Psychology, 46, 398-401.

Heilbrun, A. B., & Friedberg, L. (1991). Higher-order relationships between body-perception indices and locus of defense. Currently unpublished study.

Heilbrun, A. B., Friedberg, L., & Wydra, D. (1989). Personality underlying motivation for Type A behavior in late adolescents. Journal of Youth and Adolescence, 18, 311-319.

Heilbrun, A. B., Friedberg, L., Wydra, D., & Worobow, A. L. (1990). The female role and menstrual distress: An explanation for inconsistent evidence. Psychology of Women Quarterly, 14, 403-417.

Heilbrun, A. B., & Handfinger, A. S. (1992). The role of psychological defenses in combat-related posttraumatic stress disorder. Currently unpublished study.

Heilbrun, A. B., & Harris, A. (1986). Psychological defenses in females at-risk for anorexia nervosa: An explanation for excessive stress found in anorexic patients. International Journal of Eating Disorders, 5, 503-516.

Heilbrun, A. B., & Hausman, G. A. (1990). Perceived enhancement of body size in women sharing anorexic psychological characteristics: The role of self-preoccupation. International Journal of Eating Disorders, 9, 283-291.

Heilbrun, A. B., & Karp, J. F. (1992). Deficient problem-solving skills as an explanation of Type A motive conflict in competition. Currently unpublished study.

Heilbrun, A. B., & Lozman, R. (1991). Body-image distortion and dis-attention to internal stimulation: Alternative or common anorectic risk factors? Currently unpublished study.

Heilbrun, A. B., & Mofield, K. (1991). Motives for competition in stress-prone Type As. Currently unpublished study.

Heilbrun, A. B., & Mulqueen, C. M. (1987). The second androgyny: A proposed revision in adaptive priorities for college women. Sex Roles, 17, 187-207.

Heilbrun, A. B., & Norbert, N. (1972). Self-regulatory behavior in skid-row alcoholics. Quarterly Journal of Studies on Alcohol, 33, 989-998.

Heilbrun, A. B., Palchanis, N., & Friedberg, E. (1986). Self-report measurement of Type A behavior: Toward refinement and improved prediction. Journal of Personality Assessment, 50, 525-539.

Heilbrun, A. B., & Pepe, V. (1985). Awareness of cognitive defenses and stress management. British Journal of Medical Psychology, 58,

9-17.

Heilbrun, A. B., & Putter, L. D. (1986). Preoccupation with stereotyped sex role differences, ideal body weight, and stress in college women showing anorexic characteristics. International Journal of Eating Disorders, 5, 1035-1049.

Heilbrun, A. B., & Renert, D. (1986). Type A behavior, cognitive defense, and stress. Psychological Reports, 58, 447-456.

Heilbrun, A. B., & Renert, D. (1988). Psychological defenses and menstrual distress. British Journal of Medical Psychology, 61, 219-230.

Heilbrun, A. B., & Schwartz, H. L. (1979). Defensive style and performance on objective personality measures. Journal of Personality Assessment, 43, 517-525.

Heilbrun, A. B., & Schwartz, H. L. (1980). Self-esteem and self-reinforcement in men alcoholics: An explanation of a paradox. Journal of Studies on Alcohol, 41, 1134-1142.

Heilbrun, A. B., Tarbox, A. R., & Madison, J. K. (1979). Cognitive structure and behavioral regulation in alcoholics. Journal of Studies on Alcohol, 40, 387-400.

Heilbrun, A. B., & Witt, N. (1990). Distorted body image as a risk factor in anorexia nervosa: Replication and clarification. Psychological Reports, 66, 407-416.

Heilbrun, A. B., & Worobow, A. L. (1990). Attention and disordered eating behavior: II. Disattention to turbulent inner sensations as a risk factor in the development of anorexia nervosa. Psychological Reports, 66, 467-478.

Heilbrun, A. B., & Worobow, A. L. (1991). Attention and disordered eating behavior: I. Disattention to satiety cues as a risk factor in the development of bulimia. Journal of Clinical Psychology, 47, 3-9.

Heilbrun, A. B., Wydra, D., & Friedberg, L. (1989). Sex role correlates of stress-prone Type A behavior of college students. Sex Roles, 21, 433-449.

Herzberg, F. I. (1970). A study of the psychological factors in primary dysmenorrhea. Journal of Clinical Psychology, 8, 174-178.

Jenkins, C. D., Rosenman, R. H., & Zyzanski, S. J. (1974). Prediction of clinical coronary heart disease by a test for coronary-prone behavior pattern. The New England Journal of Medicine, 23, 1271-1275.

Jenkins, C. D., Zyzanski, S. J., & Rosenman, R. H. (1971). Progress toward validation of a computer-scored test for the Type A coronary-prone behavior pattern. Psychosomatic Medicine, 40, 25-43.

Jenkins, C. D., Zyzanski, S. J., Rosenman, R. H., & Cleveland, G. (1971). Association of coronary-prone behavior scores with recurrence of coronary heart disease. Journal of Chronic Diseases, 24, 601-611.

Keith, R. L., Lown, B., & Stare, F. J. (1965). Coronary heart disease and behavior patterns: An examination of method. Psychosomatic Medicine, 27, 424-434.

Kelly, J. A., Furman, W., & Young, V. (1978). Problems associated with typological measurement of sex roles and androgyny. Journal of Consulting and Clinical Psychology, 46, 1574-1576.

Kenigsberg, D., Zyzanski, S. J., Jenkins, C. D., Wardwell, W. I., & Licciardello, A. T. (1974). The coronary-prone behavior pattern in hospitalized patients with and without coronary heart disease. Psychosomatic Medicine, 36, 344-351.

Kestenberg, J. S. (1961). Menarche. In S. Lorand & H. Schneer (Eds.), Adolescents' psychoanalytic approach to problems and therapy (pp. 19-50). New York: Paul B. Hoeber.

Kissileff, H. R., Thornton, J., & Becker, E. (1982). A quadratic equation adequately describes the cumulative food intake curve in man. Appetite, 3, 255-272.

Lazarus, R. S., & Folkman, S. (1984). Stress, appraisal, and coping. New York: Springer.

Logue, C. M., & Moos, R. (1986). Perimenstrual symptoms: Prevalence and risk factors. Psychosomatic Medicine, 48, 388-414.

Madison, J. K. (1983). Memory for interpersonal information. Doctoral dissertation, Emory University, Atlanta, Georgia.

Markus, H. (1977). Self-schemata and processing information about the self. Journal of Personality and Social Psychology, 35, 63-78.

Matthews, K. (1982). Psychological perspectives on the Type A behavior pattern. Psychological Bulletin, 91, 293-323.

McGovern, S. (1988). The value of thinness in females: Age and sex-role factors. Doctoral dissertation, Emory University, Atlanta, Georgia.

Mednick, S. A., & Schulsinger, F. (1970). Factors related to breakdown in children at high risk for schizophrenia. In M. Roff & D. F. Ricks (Eds.), Life history research in psychopathology (pp. 51-93). Minneapolis: University of Minnesota Press.

Meltzer, L. (1974). The aging female: A study of attitudes toward aging and self-concept held by pre-menopausal, menopausal, and post-menopausal women. Dissertation Abstracts International, 35, 1055-B.

Menninger, K. (1939). Somatic correlations with the unconscious repudiation of femininity in women. Journal of Nervous and Mental Disease, 89, 514-527.

Mills, C. J. (1983). Sex-typing and self-schemata effects on memory and response latency. Journal of Personality and Social Psychology, 45, 163-172.

Moos, R. (1968). The development of a menstrual distress questionnaire. Psychosomatic Medicine, 30, 853-867.

Moos, R. (1969). Typology of menstrual cycle symptoms. American Journal of Obstetrics and Gynecology, 103, 390-403.

Moos, R. (1986). Menstrual Distress Questionnaire manual. Los Angeles: Western Psychological Services.

Morse, C. A., & Dennerstein, L. (1988). The factor structure of symptom reports in premenstrual syndrome. Journal of Psychosomatic Research, 32, 93-98.

Murray, H. (1938). Explorations in personality. New York: Oxford University Press.

Nideffer, R. (1973). Preliminary manual for the Test of Attentional and Interpersonal Styles. The University of Rochester, Rochester, New York.

Nix, J., & Lohr, J. M. (1981). Relationship between sex, sex-role characteristics, and coronary-prone behavior in college students. Psychological Reports, 48, 737-744.

Nowicki, S., Jr., & Duke, M. P. (1974). A locus of control scale for college as well as noncollege adults. Journal of Personality Assessment, 38, 136-137.

Olds, D. E., & Shaver, P. (1980). Masculinity, femininity, academic performance, and health: Further evidence concerning the androgyny controversy. Journal of Personality, 48, 323-341.

Paige, K. (1973). Women learn to sing the menstrual blues. Psychology Today, 7, 41-46.

Palermo, D. S., & Jenkins, J. J. (1964). Word association norms: Grade school through college. Minneapolis: University of Minnesota Press.

Parsons, T., & Bales, R. F. (1955). Family, socialization, and interaction process. Glencoe, Ill.: Free Press.

Paulson, M. J. (1956). Psychological concomitants of premenstrual tension. Doctoral dissertation, University of Kansas, Lawrence, Kansas.

Peshkin, H. (1968). The duration of normal menses as a psychosomatic phenomenon. Psychosomatic Medicine, 30, 378-389.

Price, V. A. (1982). Type A behavior pattern: A model for research and practice. New York: Academic Press.

Rodin, J., Silberstein, L., & Striegel-Moore, R. (1985). Women and weight: A normative discontent. In T. B. Sonderegger (Ed.), Psychology and gender: Nebraska Symposium on Motivation, 1984, (pp. 267-307). Lincoln: University of Nebraska Press.

Robins, L. N. (1966). Deviant children grownup: A psychiatric and sociological study of sociopathic personality. Baltimore: Williams & Wilkins.

Rosenman, R. H. (1978). The interview method of assessment of the coronary-prone behavior pattern. In T. M. Dembroski, S. M. Weiss, J. L. Shields, S. G. Hayes, & M. Feinleib (Eds.), Coronary-prone behavior (pp. 55-69). New York: Springer-Verlag.

Rosenman, R. H., Friedman, M., & Straus, R. (1964). A predictive study of coronary heart disease: The Western Collaborative Group Study. Journal of the American Medical Association, 189, 15-26.

Rosenman, R. H., Friedman, M., Straus, R., Wurm, M., Jenkins, C. D., & Messinger, H. B. (1966). Coronary heart disease in the western collaborative group study: A follow-up experience of two years. Journal of the American Medical Association, 195, 86-92.

Rotter, J. (1966). Generalized expectancies for internal versus external control of reinforcement. Psychological Monographs: General and Applied, 80 (whole No. 609), 1-28.

Schneider, J. F., & Schneider-Duker, M. R. (1974). Conservative attitudes and reactions to menstruation. Psychological Reports, 35, 1304.

Selye, H. (1976). The stress of life. New York: McGraw-Hill.

Sessions, P. M. (1967). Social casework treatment of alcoholics with the focus on the image of self. In R. Fox (Ed.), Alcoholism: Behavioral research, therapeutic approaches (pp. 299-320). New York: Springer.

Shader, R. I., & Ohly, J. I. (1970). Premenstrual tension, femininity, and sexual drive. Medical Aspects of Human Sexuality, 4, 42.

Shaffer, D. R. (1988). Social and personality development (2nd ed.). Pacific Grove, CA: Brooks/Cole.

Shainess, N. (1961). A re-evaluation of some aspects of femininity through a study of menstruation. Comprehensive Psychiatry, 2, 10-26.

Slade, P. (1982). Towards a functional analysis of anorexia nervosa and bulimia nervosa. British Journal of Clinical Psychology, 21, 167-179.

Slade, P. D. (1985). A review of body-image studies in anorexia nervosa and bulimia nervosa. Journal of Psychiatric Research, 19, 255-265.

Slade, P., & Jenner, F. A. (1980). Attitudes toward female roles, aspects of menstruation and complaining of menstrual symptoms. British Journal of Social and Clinical Psychology, 19, 109-113.

Slade, P. D., & Russell, G. F. M. (1973). Awareness of body dimensions in anorexia nervosa: Cross-cultural and longitudinal studies. Psychological Medicine, 3, 188-199.

Smith, G. P., & Gibbs, J. (1979). Postpandrial satiety. Progress in Psychobiology and Physiological Psychology, 18, 179-242.

Spence, J. T., Helmreich, R., & Stapp, J. (1973). A short version of the Attitude Towards Women scale (AWS). Bulletin of the Psychonomic Society, 2, 219-220.

Spence, J. T., Helmreich, R., & Stapp, J. (1975). Ratings of self and peers on sex role attributes and their relation to self-esteem and conceptions of masculinity and femininity. Journal of Personality and Social Psychology, 32, 29-39.

Spero, J. R. (1968). A study of the relationship between selected functional menstrual disorders and interpersonal conflict. Doctoral dissertation, New York University, New York, New York.

Squires, R. L., & Kagan, D. M. (1985). Sex-role and eating behaviors among college women. International Journal of Eating Disorders, 4, 459-548.

Tarbox, A. R. (1979). Self-regulation and sense of competence in men alcoholics. Journal of Studies on Alcohol, 40, 860-867.

Teghtsoonian, M., Becker, E., & Edelman, B. (1981). A psychophysical analysis of perceived satiety: Its relation to consummatory behavior and degree of overweight. Appetite, 2, 217-229.

Whitehouse, A. M., Freeman, C. P. L., & Annadale, A (1988). Body size estimation in anorexia nervosa. British Journal of Psychiatry, 153 (supp. 2), 23-26.

Williams, J. E., & Best, D. L. (1982). Measuring sex stereotypes: A thirty-nation study. Beverly Hills, CA: Sage.

Woods, N. F. (1985). Relationship of socialization and stress to premenstrual symptoms, disability, and menstrual attitudes. <u>Nursing Research</u>, <u>34</u>, 145-149.

Woods, D. J., & Launius, A. L. (1979). Type of menstrual discomfort and psychological masculinity in college women. <u>Psychological Reports</u>, <u>44</u>, 257-258.

Author Index

Subject Index

About the Author

Alfred B. Heilbrun Jr. received the Ph.D. degree from the University of Iowa in 1954 and served on that university's psychology faculty from 1956 to 1965. He was awarded diplomate status in 1960 by the American Board of Professional Psychology with a speciality in clinical psychology. Dr. Heilbrun joined the faculty of Emory University in 1965 where he directed the clinical psychology training program, the university counseling service, and the community-oriented Psychological Center. Dr. Heilbrun was awarded the Walter Klopfer award from the Society for Personality Assessment in 1991 for distinguished contribution to the literature of personality assessment, and that year retired from Emory University as Distinguished Research Professor of Psychology.